THE MIRACLE THAT HEALS

THE
MIRACLE
THAT
HEALS

BY

David Holland

CROYDON HOUSE

8365 N.E. 2ND AVENUE

MIAMI 38, FLORIDA

Library of Congress catalog card number 56-10263

Manufactured in the United States of America
American Book–Stratford Press, Inc., New York

1109963

FOREWORD

IN EVERY AGE throughout humanity's struggle for survival thinkers have risen above the darkness to proclaim gleams of the truth. These noble characters, holding high the torch of enlightenment, strode not only across the pages of Scripture, but through much of our early and modern literature as well. Never before has the subject of metaphysics, the philosophy of true existence first expounded seriously by Jesus, been presented to so great a host of earnest seekers after the truth as in this twentieth century.

Truth stands alone on its merit, making no compromise with, nor desiring any support from, error; for truth is the substance of God's creation, while error is a misapprehension of it. Truth destroys everything unlike itself in the ratio that its light dawns upon comprehension. This is so because both truth and its antipode, error, have their abode solely in consciousness. They can abide in no other place.

Man has an inherent right to health, happiness, abundance and eternal life, and it is his *misapprehension* of these divine gifts from God that keeps him from fully expressing them. A radical change in his thinking must therefore come about before he is able to break the illusory chains of gross materialism that bind him to his own erring thoughts.

Jesus, perhaps, was the most noteworthy person whose

spiritual insight into the reality of God's kingdom has borne much fruit in behalf of mankind, yet comparatively few have the least understanding of what his teachings imply. The multiplicity of theological beliefs and their divergent interpretations attest this verity.

The author, in his endeavor to elucidate on so profound a theme as the truth, has foregone any attempt to bring this infinite subject within the bounds of chronological order. This position is obvious when one considers the many approaches necessary to clearly interpret a single phase of truth. Hence, he has written on this stupendous topic as, and in the order that, the light of spontaneity entered his consciousness. Such a work is not peculiarly adaptable to the established formula, nor is it desirable.

It is not without a definite purpose that a number of passages from the Scriptures, as well as significant extracts from the author's own commentaries, are reiterated in differing aspects. It is only by throwing a recurring light on the many facets of such an exposition that the reader can fairly obtain a grasp of its unfoldment, while it is not infrequently that a clarity of understanding may come through but a single facet alone.

Language, man's invention to express his thoughts, is hardly adequate in revealing spiritual impressions, inasmuch as one is compelled to make use of physical interpretations to explain spiritual conceptions. Thus, when defining the spiritual, material pictures intrude upon the mental vision to blot out the divine reality. This is the nature of material sense; and it is only by constant repetition of the spiritual exposition, in various presentations, that the real painting of Spirit can be effectively impressed and retained in the mind.

There is nothing difficult in comprehending metaphysics. It is as susceptible to reason as is any question giving impulse to inquiry. But, like all scientific knowledge, the truth needs to be pondered, weighed, and carefully analyzed. It requires dwelling upon to clearly see the gaping disparities that exist between reality and error.

The truth demands study and application no less than the arts, mathematics, engineering, or any other branch of learning. This is particularly so owing to the fact that humanity for centuries on end has been influenced by the engulfing currents of superstition, ignorance, fear, credulity, sorcery, bigotry, and the whole range of human errors down to present-day prejudices and dogmatism.

Man clings obstinately to the fallacies of existence for the reason that they have been inculcated in him from the cradle. This affection for error can be dissolved only with the solvent of truth. Since everything erroneous resides solely in your mind, it is here alone that the transformation must take place.

Although a single perusal of this volume should unfold numerous gleams of the truth in your consciousness, it is only by giving it diligent study and application that truth's greater glow will take possession of your thinking, lift you into the full bloom of health, and bring you into dominion over both yourself and the world you live in.   D. H.

THE MIRACLE THAT HEALS is *not* intended to be a religious discourse, but rather a philosophic and scientific approach to the truth of being. Wholly inspirational in character, this work is brought forth primarily to reveal the practical utilisation of *truth* in human welfare.

"If the body is to be well, you must begin by curing the mind."

—*Socrates*

THE MIRACLE THAT HEALS

CHAPTER I

PERFECT HEALTH is man's greatest possession. He treasures it above all things, yet nothing perhaps is so little understood and abused as is his physical well-being. Whenever he looks outside of himself to preserve it, or to regain it for that matter, his endeavors are encumbered with fearful odds.

Poor mortal! Little is he aware that perfect health is wholly within himself. He needs only to realize this. To embrace it. Enjoy it.

Jesus, the master metaphysician, discovered the Creator and *all* that He created within himself. This revelation was passed on to all posterity when he said, concisely:

"The kingdom of God is within you."

This was not an idle statement. Nor was it the promise of some reward to be realized after death. On the contrary, it was the truth of conscious, practical being that he had made known, a present reality that can be evidenced *here* and *now*.

This disclosure intimated dominion over everything upon the earth, and the strength and ability to fully utilize this mighty power. Indeed, this richest of all heritages is a divine birthright which God has given to every man without reservation.

Think of it! A blessing so great that you are scarcely able to conceive, much less embrace, the smallest part of it. And this is the inexhaustible domain that inherently is within every one of us.

How unavailing then for man to look outside of himself for that which already is within him by mandate of his Creator. Little wonder that he can neither preserve, nor restore, his health whenever he looks elsewhere for it than within himself.

A mere conscious gleam of this healing truth, although it may linger with you but for a fleeting moment, is often sufficient to make you instantly well, notwithstanding that you may be the victim of the most dreaded disease, and on the threshold of death itself.

Did not Paul say:

"For the word of God is quick, and powerful, and sharper than any twoedged sword."?

Health, be it good or bad, is your individual mental state. It has no other tangibility nor substance. It exists solely within your mind. You, alone, unwittingly give health its bloom and vigor no less than its morbid symptoms and impotence.

There is but *one* way to prove the truth: can you demonstrate it? Heal yourself? Live happily? Unless you can consciously feel and see yourself a part of truth, and responsive to it, all the blind beliefs of prevailing doctrine will never bring you in rapport with it.

To consider for a passing moment the profound implication of the Master's revealing statement,

"The kingdom of God is within you,"

is to become pleasantly aware that you possess the divine power to express the evidence of its import.

This promising declaration is indeed more than just a beautifully-couched phrase to lull the disquieted spirit. It is the *truth*. Not only of the Master's day. But the truth *today*. The truth *forever*. This power is in you and me, and the Eskimo in the frozen North fishing through the ice for his daily sustenance.

Countless millions of sermons have been preached, published and debated from pulpit, press and street-corner on this Scriptural passage, and virtually all have circumvented its true application. Of the hundreds of religious systems spread over the earth, there are equally as many conflicting interpretations of this significant citation.

And why has this been so?

Manifestly to perpetuate the dogmatic authority handed down to these hundreds of denominations from their respective church founders.

It must therefore be apparent that those responsible for all these discourses, propagation and controversies never truly discovered for *themselves* the deific design underlying this Biblical utterance. They merely had conformed their thought to sectarian doctrine. For nearly two thousand years this revelation has been somewhat of a paradox into which scarcely any ecclesiastic or layman dared venture beyond canonical boundaries; all of which is clearly evident, inasmuch as it involved sheer speculation from which one could hardly extricate himself.

"The kingdom of God is within you"

has no ambiguous meaning, but rather is it as understandable as any literal combination of words made up for a child's comprehension. But so long as its true sense is associated with materiality, the substance of matter, you at once lose the very essence and spirit of its nature, and wander instead into a maze of darkness.

This darkness, or material existence, is the *void* which has no abiding place in God's infinite creation.

If the kingdom of God is within us, as Jesus assures us it is, then surely we have the power to cast out, as he had, disease, poverty, evil and death, and in their place experience health, abundance, goodness and everlasting life. Did he not likewise say:

"He that believeth on me, the works that I do shall he do also; and greater works than these shall he do."?

There was no ambiguity whatever in that statement. It admits of no other interpretation. And he was addressing you and me, no less than his disciples, and Lee Wong in the back country of China, the peasant Giuseppe in Italy, and the Ubangi tribesman in the wilds of Africa. To be sure, he was addressing every image and likeness of God on the face of the earth.

Do you believe this?

Here is the measure of your faith.

Jesus was not alluding to any *hereafter*. He was speaking of *now*, the ever-present. He always spoke only in terms of the eternal, never in the fleeting dimensions of time. Paul substantiated this fact when he said:

"Behold, *now* is the accepted time; behold, *now* is the day of salvation."

Time is but a mortal limiting rod, and God knows nothing of it. It is a millstone around man's neck, a pillory to which he has unwittingly shackled himself. *Now* is ever, always.

Let us look intelligently into the matter, and reason together.

It is self-evident that we must have a base for our thought, for only on such a foundation could the source and continuity of our being rest; and this base, common sense tells us, is God. The budding tree, the rising sun, the unfolding petals of a rose, the precision-like activities of the universe, the song of a thrush, all attest this verity. Must we look farther?

Every renowned astronomer, physicist, logician and savant subscribes to the following affirmation:

"Everything in the cosmos is perfect and harmonious in structure, arrangement and activity; it is only man's concept of it that is imperfect and discordant."

This arresting truth by no means is confined alone to the planetary system in the outer reaches of the universe, but to each idea and action on the earth, infinitesimal as it might be, including man himself.

This directs us naturally to the age-old question that always has perplexed mankind: what *is* God?

From Genesis to Revelation we are told that He is Spirit; and this definition is generally accepted by all humanity. That is to say, God is not constituted, as we believe we are, of flesh and blood.

Here it becomes necessary to probe into the very quintessence of Spirit if we are to see for ourselves what It actually is. Consequently, if we are Spirit's image and likeness, we are It's derivative. And unless we fairly learn the true *substance* of this derivative, we shall never know what God is, nor His creation, of which we are sensibly cognizant.

Surely this should be a reasonable basis from which to proceed.

Every dictionary, or similar authority, is agreed that Spirit is the direct opposite of matter, or anything constituted of a physical nature. Reasoning from this principle, inasmuch as we are the image and likeness of Spirit, it would be safe here to discard matter from any further consideration in our logic. But, of course, we shall defer doing this until first we are thoroughly convinced that materiality is a bald imposition on our faculties of awareness.

Notwithstanding all the convictions to the contrary, man is not a material entity despite the fact that he appears to be compounded of matter. That this is so, Paul stated, explicitly:

"Ye are *not* in the flesh, but in the Spirit. They which are the children of the flesh, these are *not* the children of God."

This point could hardly be set forth plainer. And so, from here on, we are obliged to resort to reason, a rather sound judge, tempered with the wisdom of the oracles and sages of the past, to whom a mystified humanity has ever looked for light and guidance.

Spirit, if It is not matter, obviously must be divine awareness; or, to be more specific, divine consciousness, or mind. It is *knowing*. Or to be right back where we began, mere thought. And that alone explains what God truly is, the wellspring of thought. He is awareness, consciousness, mentality, knowing.

He is *not* material substance, nor contained in any physical form; and of that, without serious question, we are universally agreed.

It is well to quote, in our search for the truth, out of the first chapter of Genesis:

"God created man in His own image, in the image of God created He him; male and female created He them."

If man is God's derivative, and made of His substance, he then must be constructed purely of spiritual consciousness, in the image and likeness of his Creator. Seeing that God is fundamentally *thought,* so must His image likewise be *thought,* as must His entire creation. Image exists solely in mind, never in matter. Consequently, man, too, is wholly awareness, consciousness, mentality, knowing. Clearly stated, man is the image, or reflection, of God's consciousness.

A child could come to no other conclusion.

Where then comes the bald imposition on our perceptive faculties that we are material beings?

Paul also said:

"Flesh and blood cannot inherit the kingdom of God."

This declaration has been reiterated in one way or another throughout the entire length of the Bible; and it should be plain to the least discerning mind that man, whom God created in His image and likeness, definitely *cannot* be flesh and blood, or any other material substance, if he is spiritually endowed with His kingdom.

And let it not be assumed that this kingdom is inherited in death. Indeed, it can only be realized in life, *now.* Jesus made this point clear:

"God is not the God of the dead, but of the living."

The kingdom of God, His creation, which the Master said was within you, is similarly reflected, as is your own image-identity, through the medium of awareness, consciousness, mentality, knowing. Nothing supposedly material outside of yourself can impart a conscious impression.

Let us look at this important point in another light.

We are generally agreed that God's creation is the result of His own making, and that everything in and comprising it is subject to His authority and law. Plausibly, it cannot be a material creation if God is Spirit. And if all was *void*, or nothingness, before the universe was cast into existence, from where could its Creator reasonably obtain the myriad components and masses of materiality out of which to make the infinite numbers of planets and constellations constituting the cosmos, of which the earth is but a grain of matter in comparison?

It is very well to say that everything was made out of chaos at the mere word, or command, of God; and there it was, a material universe, physically constructed to its final component. But ask yourself, in all candor, is there not something definitely illogical about such a creation that instantly moves your matured intelligence to question it?

Or would it not be more likely, and far more beautiful and consistent with reason, to believe His creation was made solely out of His own substance, His consciousness?

If God is Spirit, and that is *all* there really is, or was, from the beginning, then everything that He had made inevitably must be spiritual. Everything is conceived in Spirit, formed in Spirit, dwells in Spirit, and is sustained by Spirit.

We erroneously invert the real, and call the inversion

material and genuine when it is merely an illusion of the
human senses that we perceive. This explains why we have
so much discord and pain in both ourselves and the so-
called physical world about us.

Paul makes this rather plain:

> **"For he that soweth to his flesh shall of the flesh reap cor-
> ruption; but he that soweth to the Spirit shall of the
> Spirit reap life everlasting."**

Everything that man sees spiritually, for indeed there is
no other power whereby to see, his inverted sense fancies
it as being constructed of matter. And so it is with all his
other senses, hearing, feeling, tasting and smelling.

Whatever exists *must* be spiritual, the conscious ideas
and activities comprising the creation; and this God holds
eternally and completely in His mind.

There is *nothing* outside of His mind, be it substance,
space or time.

If, as Jesus so confidently assures us,

> **"The kingdom of God is within you,"**

and me, and everyone else upon the face of the earth, we
then essentially must reflect that which is in God's mind.
This includes the whole cosmos, no less than all the activities upon our own planet, for the entirety of creation is the
kingdom which He embraces in His consciousness. It is
self-evident that He did not make a separate kingdom for
each individual, but rather *one* creation for all individuals, and it is this *one* kingdom which each one of us reflects, in consciousness alone.

To illustrate: the sun is a fixed idea, or thought, in the
mind of God, and is reflected to all of us spiritually, or

mentally, through the medium of consciousness; but we, misapprehending the true substance of God's idea, interpret the sun as a physical or material object, when in reality it is evidence of His thought transmitted to us consciously. The sun's heat, light and rotation similarly are mental manifestations.

And here it is well to impress upon ourselves that an image, likeness or reflection, whether of ourselves or an inanimate object, is not the original. That is wholly the God-conception. An image is rather a consciously visible representation of the original, as you might behold your own likeness before a mirror. This divine marvel of reflection includes everything in the creation, man, tree, bird, sunshine, rain, and the palatial liner afloat on the bosom of the sea.

God's mind is the unbounded sanctum wherein *all* the ideas and activities of creation, including man, abide.

To put it in still another light, if

"The kingdom of God is within you,"

it must be His spiritual consciousness alone which you embody. Surely a material kingdom could never be implanted in you, for where and how could you contain it? Not in your supposedly material body, which you are disposed to believe is your true self.

The fact is you infold God's kingdom only in your consciousness. For that is what you, your body, and everything within the scope of your senses really are, God's reflected ideas in consciousness. There is *nothing* else but divinely conscious ideas throughout the entire gamut of His creation.

Inasmuch as both you and the kingdom are spiritual

realities in God's mind, *everything* obviously must be made solely out of, and subsist in, the substance of His consciousness.

How else could one possibly be the beneficiary of God's kingdom if not from the standpoint of the mental?

Man is the image and likeness of Spirit, not matter, and inherently must exist as Spirit's offspring, or spiritual derivative. He does not live outside of God, but *in* Him. In His consciousness.

This is the *truth* about man. It is exactly what Jesus was endeavoring to impress upon the Jews in the temple, when he declared:

"Ye shall know the truth, and the truth shall make you free."

Free of what?

Obviously free of the erring beliefs, in human consciousness, that deface and enfeeble mankind's so-called physical bodies, and bind and chain them to disease, poverty, evil and death. Yes, free man with the potency of truth from the fettering belief that he is the material image of, and a detached entity from, a God that is admitted to be Spirit.

Is this too much for you to accept?

If so, be not discouraged. Truth is a stranger where error predominates. On the evening of the Feast of the Passover, while teaching his humble disciples, the Master said:

"I have yet many things to say unto you, but ye cannot bear them now."

Think of it! The wealth of unfoldment and power Jesus was constrained to keep pent up within himself.

And why?

Because even the apostles were inclined to question the truth which he taught. Its simple philosophy seemed to border on the fanciful.

Perhaps you, too, are not able to bear this truth either.

Whatever your quandary or reservations, truth goes sweeping on down the corridors of time notwithstanding.

So here we are, standing at the fork in the road that leads to truth and error. Which will you follow?

This is indeed a momentous decision, so be not hasty in choosing wisely.

And while you take counsel with yourself, it might be well to direct these significant words to you that Jesus addressed to his disciples as he sat in a ship by the seaside:

"Verily I say unto you, that many prophets and righteous men have desired to see those things which ye see, and have not seen them; and to hear those things which ye hear, and have not heard them."

CHAPTER II

THIS IS a golden age for those that dare break away from material precedents of the past and think for themselves. To such as these, the enlightening influence of reason will direct their footsteps and be a yardstick for progress. There is absolutely *no* power nor existence outside of consciousness. Whatever you choose to conceive, externalize into form, and finally place into operation to fulfil the ends of your purpose, must wholly take place in mind.

There is this striking difference between God's thinking and the thinking of mortals or fleshly beings: God's thoughts are creative ideas and eternal verities, while a mortal's thoughts are mental misconceptions of His ideas, and therefore basically erroneous and perishable. This is so because everything appears structurally material to us. Consequently, we believe ourselves to be material flesh and bones, and contain within this formation of seeming protoplasm a self-sufficient existence.

Of this erroneous belief, Isaiah declared:

"Cease ye from man, whose breath is in his nostrils: for wherein is he to be accounted of?"

This stricture of mortal man, whose appearance is simply an imposture of God's image and likeness, bears out the fallacy of our beliefs. This supposedly real man, whom we assume to be material, is nothing more than a *mental* concept of what we have miscreated.

Knowing, instead, that we are indissolubly spiritual, if we are the image and likeness of Spirit, our thoughts naturally must reflect the eternal character of God. The sum total of His ideas constitutes His infinite creation, and man is one of the ideas, as is the blade of grass, the honeybee, and the Pleiades which sprinkle the heavens above.

According to St. John:

> **"All things were made by Him; and without Him was not anything made that was made."**

That should be clear enough. Anything that was made without Him definitely is perishable, and short-lived. It cannot be real nor eternal. Consequently, it must be *illusion.*

It is not necessary, as humanity is inclined to believe, that God cast His ideas in clay; for when He declared them ideas, they instantly became substantial and clothed in the beauty and permanency of Spirit. Only misconceived thought would defile God's ideas with matter.

Of the illusion of flesh and bones, Job said:

> **"Man that is born of a woman is of few days, and full of trouble."**

Such a man obviously is *not* the image and likeness of God.

Indeed, man does not have to die first to learn the true nature about God and himself. God's man *never* dies. He is as eternal as his Father. The truth exists *now*, and there is no hereafter. The belief of a hereafter is error, evil. It is utter illusion.

All this outworn doctrine of a hereafter is equivalent to a confession of ignorance as to the true facts. We have no less an authority for this than Jesus himself, who said, rather plainly:

"This is life eternal, that they might know Thee the only true God."

He made no mention of a future life. He was speaking of *this* life as being eternal. Where then comes the hereafter?

And if this disclosure should fall short of satisfying your skepticism, the Master put it still another way:

"If a man keep my saying, he shall never see death."

Man is the image of God's consciousness, and that is all there is to him. There is no more, except it be an illusion that he is matter. And here it might be well to state that God's consciousness, or your own, is not confined in a human form of protoplasm, much less a skull. To believe so is simply to stretch the illusion.

The only hell or hereafter there is, or can be, is in the belief that man is a physical entity, adequate unto himself. And of this entity, it is well foretold:

"For dust thou art, and unto dust shalt thou return."

This is the man that is made up from unequal parts of phosphorus, calcium, carbon, lime, among other things, plus ten gallons of water; all of which can be purchased at current rates of less than a dollar.

Is this combination of material ingredients man? The man whom God made in His image and likeness? And can this mixture of matter produce life? Intelligence? Foresight?

The real man is spiritual, and can *never* be compounded of material substance. He lives in God's mind, as one of His ideas, the most favored one, and this alone confutes matter as having existence.

Nothing can separate this man from God, and Paul confirms this fact:

> "Neither death, nor life . . . nor things present, nor things to come . . . nor any other creature, shall be able to separate us from the love of God."

The question naturally arises:

> "What then is all this materiality that is my body and the world around me; and my friend, John Brown, that I saw buried in the ground only yesterday?"

It is illusion, all of it, notwithstanding that it has the familiar appearances of reality, color, symmetry, firmness, and answers to all the phenomena of the five physical senses.

Here we are confronted with the greatest of all mysteries ever to challenge human thought: is matter real or is it merely an illusion? This is the poser which Jesus specifically alluded to when he said:

> "Ye shall know the truth, and the truth shall make you free."

Not only the Master, but all the foremost personages of the Bible have unmistakably intimated the unreality of matter, as have the world's most celebrated philosophers, oracles and thinkers. Indeed, God never made *anything* mortal. Everything that He had made was immortal.

This is the high point of our discourse, the key to all truth, the secret to healing the discordant body. With this light of understanding dawning in good time upon your receptive thought, you, too, shall know the truth to which Jesus alluded, and this truth shall make you free.

Spirituality and materiality do not combine to make man, much as you are disposed to believe so. They have no attraction one for the other. This is the great error that has beset man from time immemorial, and it is this blindness to truth that has made him diseased, evil, inadequate, and subject to death. And so long as he continues to entertain this error of belief in his heart, he will inevitably manifest the fruits of its falsity in his experience.

It is just such a man, without the divine quality, of whom Paul had reference, when he said:

"Flesh and blood cannot inherit the kingdom of God."

This should satisfy the most skeptical that the kingdom is not material, but spiritual, divine consciousness. Like man, it has not the slightest element of materiality in its construction.

Or perhaps you might better understand the Master's outspoken disdain for the material man:

"Ye are of your father the devil, and the lusts of your father ye will do. He was a murderer from the beginning, and abode not in the truth, because there is no truth in him. When he speaketh a lie, he speaketh of his own: for he is a liar, and the father of it. And because I tell you the truth, ye believe me not."

Do *you* believe this truth which Jesus set forth? Agree with his scathing condemnation of man supposedly made from matter? This man born of the flesh? This lie that can only multiply itself in falsity?

This is the man whom Paul says can never inherit the kingdom of God.

And why?

Because such a man is simply an illusion of belief. A nonentity to be exact. He is evil. It is idolatry to believe he can be anything else.

To be sure, Jesus was not rebuking your father made in the image and likeness of God, but his mistaken belief that he is a material and self-sufficient entity capable of procreating material life. For it is out of this deep-seated error that the lesser ones take root, bringing forth their kind in the fruits of added falsity, lust, disease, and all the evils of material thinking.

This is an important point to grasp, and retain in thought. There is no truth in this man. He alone is the devil, evil. His progeny speaketh this lie in turn, and likewise become the fathers of it.

You do not lose your individuality by accepting the fact that you are solely spiritual consciousness, and nothing more. Indeed, you come more vividly into its full realization.

The material body, that you are inclined to believe is you, only appears to be material is all; and where this body appears to be is, conversely, your spiritual body, or true self. This latter state is the image or witness, which you are, of God.

Your so-called material body is merely a physical illusion. And that is what gets sick and suffers and dies, the illusion, *never* your spiritual body, which is the conscious reflection or identity of God, and the *only* true body that you have.

God is perfect. He never gets sick and suffers and dies,

and it is He whom you reflect in His likeness. It is obvious that a material man cannot be the image of God and yet mirror disease and inharmony.

Everything that you see which seems to you to be material is, in fact, nothing more than an *image* of misconstrued thought in your consciousness. You can discard what appears to be you, leaving only the image or reflection which you are of God, and you actually will part with nothing. The only thing you can possibly discard is a *belief* of a material body that does not, and cannot, exist in reality, but is simply an illusion of thought.

This picture of material belief will disappear from your consciousness in the ratio that you see the purely spiritual image of yourself that is the reflection of God. It is much the same as any mathematical, or other, error giving place to a correct solution.

You can never discard anything that God had made because it is eternal. Your conception of a material body, or thing, which is not God-created and consequently not real, lives only in the realm of your erring thought, and this alone is what you discard. A belief of something that merely seems to be real but definitely is without the least scintilla of substantiality.

Only that which God created has substance. It is the substance of His consciousness, and therefore substantial.

God's whole creation, including you, is conceived and forged solely out of His consciousness, the only substance existent out of which He possibly could make it. Moreover, it is sustained with all its multitudinous activities in His mind. It could not exist outside of His mind, because there can be *nothing* outside of His awareness.

If we were actually material creatures, we could never

exist in a state of mind. Matter living in mind is a self-evident absurdity. The truth is we live in the mind of God as spiritual, or mental, entities. Paul clearly confirms this verity:

"In Him we live, and move, and have our being."

All that *is* is in God's mind. You, and the stars, and the tiny green shoot that thrusts itself up out of the ground to become an ear of bearded wheat, are the ideas, actualities, that exist in the mind of God; and everything in His mind is perfect, peaceful and harmonious.

You are perhaps asking yourself,

"Just what is an idea, and how can it have actual existence if nothing essentially is material to conceive and evolve it?"

An idea is purely a mental image conceived and fulfilled in the mind. It is nothing more, nor less. It has actual existence only because God made it. No one but God can make *anything* that is real; we simply reflect His ideas, or thoughts, in our consciousness is all.

That this is so, Jesus substantiates:

"The Son can do nothing of himself, but what he seeth the Father do: for what things soever He doeth, these also doeth the Son likewise."

Nothing material can be conceived and evolved. Even though you are disposed to believe in matter's existence, it could never evolve the mere shadow of an idea. God alone conceives, evolves, and objectifies *all* ideas, and this is unfolded solely in His mind. Man simply apprehends the images, or reflections, of these divine ideas through conscious receptivity.

Specifically, God's ideas and their unfoldment to man are wholly mental revelations from conception to their final utilization. Man, as the image of God, is similarly a conscious idea, and divinely endowed to receive and appreciate all His other unfolding ideas. Such conscious manifestation is the only reality of being.

Inasmuch as *all* is mind, and *in* mind, nothing can be material. Whatever man conceives other than God's ideas is illusion, evil, or erroneous thought. His material concepts have no real existence. They quickly wither and die. Of this man, and his creations, Solomon said:

"All are of the dust, and all turn to dust again."

Actually there is only *one* person in all existence, and that one is God. What appears to be the rest, including you and me, and the cosmos in general, are merely His ideas, conceived, sustained and manifested to us in their completeness in, and through, His consciousness.

That God *is* the only person, and all else is but conscious evidence of Him, Jesus makes clear to the spiritually-minded:

"That they all may be one; as thou, Father, art in me, and I in Thee, that they also may be in us . . . even as we are one."

It is fantastic to believe that God resides in some remote corner of the cosmos, and from that abode scattered His creation near and far, only to sit back as if He had separated Himself from all that which He created. But it is more extravagant still to believe that it is material.

Wherever anything might be that God had created, be it a huge planet with all its complex activities, or an invisible filament on the epidermis of a sprout, He is there in all His glory and majesty. Everything is *in* God, and there it unfolds for our availability, for He alone is the circumference of all that He had made.

God's mind is the *only* mind there is. There is none other. Man's supposed mind, which he erroneously thinks is in a pulpy formation of protoplasm called brain, is actually the image, or reflection, of God's mind; and this image is *not* confined in any material enclosure, but rather is this seeming material boundary a misapprehension of the reflection.

Both the God-created man and the material illusion are solely mental manifestations, one being reality, the other a fallacy. Neither one is constituted of matter, but wholly of consciousness. God's man is real, eternal. The material illusion is a mistaken conception of this true man and, as Job well puts it,

"Of few days, and full of trouble."

It is therefore obvious that *all* is mind, mental.

You have no self-contained mind of your own. It is absurd to believe you have. You are a complete image of God, embracing *all* His thoughts and attributes, as your image in the mirror is a complete reflection of you. You are no more the substance of materiality, as the image and likeness of God, than is the reflection of your so-called material body which you behold in the mirror.

It is of His spiritual image that Jesus alluded to, when he said:

"The kingdom of God is within you."

This is the only *you* there is.

That which appears to be you, the material body, is but a deceptive resemblance of your true counterpart.

Here is the crux of the whole matter, believing the spiritual to be material, or the two compounded as *one*. Such a belief is the precursor of all disease, adversity and misfortune. It is the foremost evil. 1109963

The belief that a mind is in your skull, that it matures and then deteriorates, can become either learned or idiotic, that pleasure and pain, health and disease, and the birth and death of matter, are all real, is simply illusion. Moreover, to believe that your brain thinks, your nerves feel, your stomach can make you irritable and suffer, is to admit that matter has intelligence and sensation.

Of course such a belief is without foundation. All the foregoing manifestations, to identify a few, are the result of your own erring beliefs, unfolding in susceptible thought. You, alone, give these several beliefs the evolving power to outline themselves, favorably or otherwise, on your supposedly material body.

Immortal man has always existed, is always perfect in health, and always independent of the *seeming* life and intelligence that is merely an illusion of matter.

Physical testimony is a lie, and the thought conceiving this testimony is the father of it, as Jesus so forcefully stated:

> **"Ye are of your father the devil, and the lusts of your father ye will do . . . . for he is a liar, and the father of it."**

A mortal is far from being God's image. He is rather a misleading appearance of it, being as he is an illusion of belief without any substance of reality. He is an erroneous thought without permanence, while God's man is the image of *truth,* and immortal. Simply stated, a mortal is merely a conscious simulation of an immortal.

The Nazarene said:

> "Believest thou not that I am in the Father, and the Father in me? The words that I speak unto you I speak not of myself: but the Father that dwelleth in me, He doeth the works. . . . Know that I am in my Father, and ye in me, and I in you."

There can be no other interpretation of this statement than the fact that there is but *one* mind, the mind of God, and we are Its images, or witnesses. And if you still are disposed to believe that you are a complete entity within yourself, this aforesaid declaration from the Master should dispel the final doubt:

> "The Son can do nothing of himself, but what he seeth the Father do: for what things soever He doeth, these also doeth the Son likewise."

Is this not the image, or reflection, repeating what the Original does? To be sure, you are that Son too. Every man, woman and child made in the image and likeness of God is His Son. Genesis confirms this:

> "God created man in His own image, in the image of God created He him; male and female created He them."

There can be no mistaking the fact that you are His Son also, no less than Jesus. The Master made no distinction between his Sonship with God and that of his fellow man; while John similarly made this point clear in his first epistle:

> "Behold, what manner of love the Father hath bestowed upon us, that we should be called the sons of God. . . . Now are we the sons of God."

And eight hundred years earlier, Hosea touched upon this subject in like manner, declaring:

"Ye are the sons of the living God."

To believe for an instant that a fleshly brain is the seat of *mind* is to detract from the dignity and omnipotence of the Creator.

CHAPTER III

IF, BY now, the mists of materiality have not yet lifted to where you can fairly see the light of truth, you need only to open wider the doors of your receptive faculties. Imbibe this priceless knowledge slowly, consider well its philosophy, and it will infallibly bring you into robust health, peace of mind, and abundance. Jesus verifies this promise:

"Seek ye first the kingdom of God; and all these things shall be added unto you."

Continue earnestly to realize that you are solely consciousness, and that you have a spiritual body that has outline, color, symmetry, beauty, and all the freshness and activity with which God, in His wisdom and power, has endowed you.

That is positively *all* there is to you, or ever has been, or ever will be. And, incidentally, it includes all the necessary poise and grace and virtue which God had so providentially conceived.

The allness of His complex creation, retained and sustained in His consciousness, is ever *one* and *now*.

Did not Jesus make this point crystal clear, when he said:

"Before Abraham was, I am."?

By the widest stretch of the imagination the Master could never have made that statement if he believed himself and the creation material. If man is one with God, as he had plainly set forth, and His creation is ever *one* and *now*, it should be rather clear that *all* has existed in the mind of God since the dawn of eternity.

Solomon puts it another way:

"I know that, whatsoever God doeth, it shall be for ever: nothing can be put to it, nor any thing taken from it. . . . That which hath been is now; and that which is to be hath already been."

Here we have it plainly stated. Why then should it seem so incredible that Jesus existed simultaneously with, if not before, Abraham?

This revelation by the Master is no less applicable to you, and to me, and the fierce Bushman living in a grass hut in the Pacific. We all are *one*, in God's mind; and His mind is never divisible, whether in substance, time or space. What appears to us otherwise is simply illusion.

We are told, in Genesis:

"The heavens and the earth were finished, and all the host of them. And on the seventh day God ended His work which He had made."

It is self-evident, if the Scriptures are to be accepted, that God was *finished* with His work of creation, and that Abraham, Jesus, and you, and I, and the fierce Bushman, were at that moment conceived and eternally cast in His mind.

We becloud the truth of being when, in our consciousness, we materialize the multiplication of God's spiritual image and likeness, and then designate these misconcep-

tions individual flesh and blood entities. Such miscreations
exist only in belief. They are merely mental manifestations of matter, or illusion.

Jesus, as the image of God, saw the glorious truth in
all its spiritual beauty; while Abraham, as the same image,
saw apparently less of it than the Master. You and I, in the
image and likeness of God, have perhaps little more than
a profound desire to seek after this truth. On the other
hand, the fierce Bushman, who similarly reflects God in His
image, in all likelihood believes only what he physically
sees, and conversely sees only that which he physically believes.

Or to put it another way, you and I, and the Bushman,
as well as Abraham and Jesus, are varying degrees of conscious expression—according to our individual understanding—of God's being.

Briefly, it is like seeing the sun's rays as beams of molten
metal, as you believe the sun itself might be; and then
eventually realizing, with the dawn of truth, that these
material rays actually are the mental reflection of God's
solar idea, inherent in His mind, and transmitted to us
through spiritual consciousness.

So does the tenacity of illusion disappear before the
light of truth through the whole pattern of matter. There
is no other solvent for materiality than truth.

All the awesome ritual and solemnity ever devised by
man, and accepted as religious belief, can never reveal one
iota of the truth that is in any way correlated to materiality. Man can only reach God, feel His presence, hear
and commune with Him, love and be led by Him, in consciousness alone.

The Master well knew, from observation of the extravagant architecture and corporeal ritualism within the synagogues, that man too often is carried away emotionally by these materialistic surroundings, and becomes blinded to the Father he normally would worship. He made this point clear, and equally emphatic, saying:

"God is a Spirit: and they that worship Him must worship Him in Spirit and in Truth."

Isaiah, clarifying this moot question, swept aside the deceptions of matter in one bold stroke:

"Thou wilt keep him in perfect peace, whose mind is stayed on Thee."

While the Psalmist sang:

"Be still, and know that I am God."

And, again, the Master looked with apparent disfavor upon all this materialistic flamboyance when he said, in his sermon on the mount:

"When thou prayest, enter into thy closet, and when thou hast shut thy door, pray to thy Father which is in secret; and thy Father which seeth in secret shall reward thee openly."

Materialism is forever silenced by these well-advised expressions.

Only by earnestly seeking God in the calm atmosphere of spiritual consciousness can you see and feel the power of His presence. This is more effectively accomplished by closing the eyes to all physical influence.

All the material symbolisms, amulets, marble edifices and canonicals on the face of the globe are without a whit of potency to move, or gain the ear of, Omnipotence. God

surely will heed the voice of the humblest soul, even
though he be a miserable derelict lost in the flotsam of
humanity, if only he will seek Him with the fulness of his
heart.

Material stone and ritualistic paraphernalia have not
this power of attraction. Such power belongs solely to spiritual consciousness, for it alone is real, substantial, eternal.

The world's renowned physical scientists and ecclesias-
tics throughout all history are more or less agreed that
materialism, in the final analysis, has no place in God's
kingdom.

The immortal St. Augustine, one of the Fathers of the
early Christian Church, said nearly sixteen hundred years
ago:

> "How, O God, didst Thou make heaven and earth? . . .
> There was no place wherein it could be made before it
> was made, that it might be; nor didst Thou hold any-
> thing in Thy hand wherewith to make heaven and earth.
> For whence couldest Thou have what Thou hadst not
> made, whereof to make anything? Therefore Thou didst
> speak and they were made, and in Thy Word Thou
> madest these things."

Surely the essence of God's Word, that made heaven and
earth and all the things therein, could hardly have been
matter, but rather His eternal ideas conceived and formed
of His own substance, consciousness, and sustained within
Himself. For St. Augustine, in his obvious bewilderment,
on looking deeper into the true nature of the heavenly
bodies, added:

> "They ceased to be what they had been, and begin to be
> what they were not."

Were these heavenly bodies actually material, they could never possibly be changed into spiritual counterparts. What this eminent Catholic bishop perceived was merely an *illusion* of material bodies change within his own consciousness. He saw the truth, substantially as Paul had inferred:

> "Look not at the things which are seen, but at the things which are not seen: for the things which are seen are temporal; but the things which are not seen are eternal."

Nearly two hundred fifty years ago the distinguished prelate of the Church of England, George Berkeley, Bishop of Cloyne, saw this truth much clearer than did St. Augustine. He declared:

> "All those bodies which compose the mighty frame of the world, have not any subsistence without a mind, that their *being* is to be perceived or known; that consequently so long as they are not actually perceived by me, or do not exist in my mind or that of any other created spirit, they must either have no existence at all, or else subsist in the mind of some Eternal Spirit; it being perfectly unintelligible, and involving all the absurdity of abstraction, to attribute to any single part of them an existence independent of a spirit. . . . All things that exist, exist only in the mind. . . . The only thing whose existence we deny is that which philosophers call matter. . . . The hardness or softness, the color, taste, warmth, figure, or suchlike qualities . . . have been shown to exist only in the mind that perceives them."

Here is the truth of being plainly set forth by an illustrious ecclesiastic, philosopher and thinker, echoing the very quintessence of reality as revealed by the world's great oracles, mentors and spiritual leaders. Matter is but dense ignorance. No man can truly understand God and himself who believes in the substantiality of a physical universe.

Of all this seeming materialism which hems us in so irrevocably on every side, Mohandas Gandhi, the ascetic Hindu leader, said:

"Daily the conviction is growing in me that God alone is real and all else is unreal. Only when you stop caring about material things do you become their master."

This universally-respected mystic was literally confirming what St. John long ago affirmed:

"Without Him was not any thing made that was made."

Philo Judaeus, a devout Alexandrian Jew, profoundly learned in the Pentateuch, and recognized as the greatest of all philosophers and writers of Hellenistic Judaism, said:

"God having determined to found a mighty state, first conceived its form in His mind, according to which form He made a world perceptible only by the intellect. He made an incorporeal heaven, and an invisible earth, and then created the incorporeal substance of water and of air, and above all He spread light, the sun; and this again was incorporeal, perceptible only to intellect. For that which is perceptible only by intellect is as far more brilliant and splendid than that which is seen, as I conceive, the sun is than darkness, or day than night, or the intellect than any other of the outward senses by which men judge. And the invisible divine reason, perceptible only by intellect, He calls the image of God. And the image of this image is that light, perceptible only by the intellect, which is the image of divine Reason."

And then this divinely inspired oracle, contemporary of Jesus and Paul, significantly concludes:

"None of those things which are perceptible to the external (material) senses is pure."

Philo Judaeus distinctly saw the great truth wherein matter is simply an illusion. Like the Master, the prophets and apostles, he had interpreted the creation as the very substance of the Creator Himself, Spirit, or the divine Intellect.

John Wesley, founder of world-wide Methodism, touching upon material substance, asserted:

"Man is not a clod of earth, a lump of clay . . . but a spirit like his Creator."

This soul-stirring clergyman was well aware that man, if he is a spirit like his Creator, must equally be as devoid of matter as He who had created him.

One of our more modern interpreters of this truth, Father John A. O'Brien, research professor of the philosophy of religion at the University of Notre Dame, made this illuminating observation:

"We now know that what constitutes practically all matter is empty space. . . . The findings of nuclear physicists sound the death knell of materialism, as an explanation of the universe and as a philosophy of life. . . . To the real scientist there is no common clay. . . . The evidence of mathematical law of a high order which atomic researchers encounter at every step convinces them of the utter inadequacy of materialism as an explanation of their invisible world."

The great thinkers since time immemorial have established the fact long before scientific inquiry that a universe of matter, including man, is a myth. Scientific inquiry has merely confirmed the discoveries of Jesus, Paul, Philo Judaeus, and a host of other divinely inspired philosophers and scholars from antiquity to present-day enlightenment.

The conviction that matter is not real, but an illusion of a material sense of things, is the absolute basis of the Master's teachings, as it was Paul's and the apostles, and all the exalted figures animating the pages of the Bible, and similar literature edifying human consciousness.

On commending Peter for giving the correct answer as to his true identity, Jesus said:

"Flesh and blood hath not revealed it unto thee, but my Father which is in heaven."

All revelation actually comes from the Father. We, His offspring, come into this spiritual knowledge only through conscious reflection.

Johannes Kepler, discoverer of the laws of planetary motion some three hundred years ago, exclaimed while gazing out upon celestial space:

"O Lord, I am thinking Thy thoughts after Thee!"

God imprints upon your consciousness His ideas, the pictures which you believe you see outside of yourself through your optic lens. He does this in color, form, density, beauty, and in numerous other qualities of expression. Hearing, feeling, tasting and smelling similarly are conveyed to you through conscious receptivity.

Physical science, or any science in fact, cannot draw a single breath without implying metaphysics in its every calculation. Materiality has neither entity nor power of *any* kind. Sensible material objects, as so-called matter is designated, are not external to the mind, but rather exist in it, and are nothing more than conscious impressions made upon it through mental action. And so it follows that weight, thickness, space, time, motion, and all other such phenomena of materiality are likewise conscious processes of physical thought.

Indeed, physicists the world over are aware that there is a line of demarcation as to how far material substance can be reduced without it dissolving into the underlying laws of reality. None will maintain that a material appearance or occurrence is independent of a higher reality than the five physical senses perceiving it.

St. Augustine had well said:

"Science is in the mind of man,"

and this incontestable truth has rung down the corridors of time through every age in the history of mankind.

Today this same verity is being reechoed. Only sheer ignorance would picture a creator forging sun, moon and stars out of an already existent mass of chaos, or raw material. Nature, whose essence is wholly spiritual consciousness, a substance far more conformable to reason than matter, refuses to accommodate herself to such physical concepts.

It is well to consider here what outstanding authorities in the physical sciences have learned from their researches into the arcanum of matter. Sir James Hopwood Jeans, professor of astronomy at Cambridge University and Princeton, and one of the more notable physicists of the world, had this to say on the subject:

"The outstanding achievement of twentieth-century physics is not the theory of relativity . . . of quanta . . . or the

> dissection of the atom with the resultant discovery that things are not what they seem; but rather is it the general recognition that we are not yet in contact with ultimate reality. . . . The universe begins to look more like a great thought than like a great machine. Mind no longer appears as an accidental intruder into the realm of matter; we are beginning to suspect that we ought rather to hail it as the creator and governor of the realm of matter. The old dualism of mind and matter . . . seems likely to disappear . . . through substantial matter resolving itself into a creation and manifestation of mind. . . . If the universe is a universe of thought, then its creation must have been an act of thought. Indeed, the finiteness of time and space almost compels us, of themselves, to picture the creation as an act of thought."

This highly-respected scholar, honored by the foremost schools on the several continents, saw deeper into the reality of the universe than merely the outline of assumed matter. He saw God as the great Architect, molding creation out of His own consciousness, the substance of His *mind*.

The eminent scientist, Charles Proteus Steinmetz, esteemed among thinking men and women everywhere for his researches in electrophysics, gives us this revealing thought:

> "Science does not and cannot show the world as it actually is with its true facts and laws, but only as it appears to us within the inherent limitations of the human mind."

Scientist, surgeon, Nobel prize-winner, and member emeritus of Rockefeller Institute of Medical Research, Dr. Alexis Carrel, states the matter even more simply:

"We love to discover in the cosmos the geometrical forms that exist in the depths of our consciousness. Geometry does not exist in the earthly world. It is in ourselves. . . . The independence of each individual from the others and from the cosmos is an illusion."

Virtually every prominent man in the fields of theology and science see eye to eye with the Master in that

"The kingdom of God is within you."

It can *never* be otherwise.

You can butt your head into insensibility against a stone wall in denial of this truth, the fact that materiality is non-existent, but you still will be what you are, solely consciousness. And all the pain and suffering that will be your lot for so abusing your head will actually have taken place in this same consciousness, although you will believe that it is your bruised head that is the focal point of pain. To be sure, the suffering is as much your *thought,* as are both the concept that provoked you to the act and the function itself of beating out your brains against the stone wall.

The whole evolvement, including your supposedly-material head and its bruised consequence, is simply a kinetoscopic picture of your thought.

The oneness of each individual with the others and the cosmos, as Dr. Carrel had pointed out, is substantiated by Jesus:

"I and my Father are one."

And then the Nazarene adds:

"That *they* may be one, as we are."

If this were not so, the fact that we are *one* with our Maker, in His consciousness, how else could it be possible for the kingdom of God to be imparted to us? And to draw out this inference further, in what other way may we have atonement with Him who created us?

The very word, atonement, implies unity; at-*one*-ment with Him. If you are not made out of the substance of which God is constituted, His consciousness, Mind, then it would be incredible to believe that you could have atonement with Him. Only like attracts like. Even the laws of materiality support this contention. Why should Spirit demand less?

Man has the power *now* to manifest the kingdom of God, but only when he realizes and understands that he is made in His image and likeness.

This image is *never* material, but a spiritual likeness of God Himself, Spirit. And here lies the momentous revelation of the truth of being, reality, while at the same time exposing the illusory appearance of matter with all its ills and pains and misadventures.

According to Genesis, God blessed man, and said:

"Have dominion over . . . every living thing that moveth upon the earth."

To enjoy this dominion man obviously must evidence the substance and power of Him who created the earth. This can be done only through the *one* Consciousness, the oneness which correlates you and me and the Australian aborigine with the Father. And unless each and every one of us can demonstrate this dominion to some appreciable extent *here* and *now*, then Jesus' assurance that the kingdom is within us is but little more than "sounding brass."

Man can never have dominion even over himself, much less the earth, so long as he believes himself to be material.

And should you be one to question the verity of the Scriptures, as a great many do, it will avail much to lay aside your doubts for a season until its truths can be demonstrated and fairly established. For unless its claims *can* be demonstrated *here* and *now*, there is no earthly excuse for the importance of the Scriptures in the first place.

On the contrary, the promises set forth in the Scriptures *can* be demonstrated in your every walk of life, whether it be to transform the sick and incurable to health, the sinful to holiness, or the destitute to abundance. Jesus has proved these truths again and again, as have his disciples, venerable mentors that have illumined the pages of history, distinguished men of profound wisdom and, not least, humble people of the soil that have had "faith as a grain of mustard seed."

It must be clearly seen, if you would successfully demonstrate these truths, that spiritual consciousness alone is the only real substance. All that which you believe is material substance, including yourself, just *seems* to be what you assume it to be, but definitely is nothing. It is a counterfeit, or a misapprehending of the true idea.

It is much the same as seeing a mirage of something either pleasant or otherwise, and then watching it disappear from before your very eyes.

Naturally you ask yourself:

"Where did it come from? And where did it go?"

To be sure, it came from nowhere as certainly as it went nowhere. It was plainly an illusion, from beginning to end, in your consciousness. The mirage was never real, because

God never made a mirage. It was a figment entirely of your *own* making. And what *you* make materially, or what rather appears to your sense of things as being material, must similarly return to dust, or nothingness.

CHAPTER IV

ARE THE first dim rays of light beginning to break through the clouds of material darkness for you?

If not, be patient. Do not become discouraged. It will all unfold naturally for you, and understandably too. It inevitably must reveal itself, for this is its express function.

It is imperative that you know the nature of materialism if you would heal yourself of disease, replace discord with harmony, and amply fulfil your daily needs. Matter is the nightmare of existence. It is the mist obscuring reality and, therefore, the exciting cause of all disorder. To see matter in its true light is the beginning of understanding.

Although you may question the teachings of Jesus, Paul and other illustrious oracles who have strewn the paths of posterity with pearls of great wisdom, perhaps you might be more readily convinced by the world's foremost physicists that matter is *not* what you believe it to be.

Indeed, you do not live in matter, but in Spirit. That this is so, Paul makes clear:

"In Him we live, and move, and have our being."

The collected ideas of creation are absolutely scientific, and all things truly scientific must have an intelligible answer for every valid question.

Anything that can be classified as science is embraced in God's law; and His kingdom is *unerring* science.

To illustrate, mathematics is the science of measuring and determining the properties and relations of quantity; but because you are unable to compute a problem based on the principle of higher calculus, it would be absurd to say that mathematics is unscientific. To find the correct solution for any quantitative problem, you need but to attune yourself with the truth of God's mathematical law.

Music, chemistry, astronomy and metaphysics, to designate a few more, are similarly scientific; for, in their inherent nature, all cause and effect are calculated without error. Wherever error enters into the picture, it is formulated human knowledge and never scientific. Science is *absolute* truth; and if it does not bring out good alone, then by this token you shall know that it has no affinity for truth, and you can discard it at once into the realm of illusion.

There is no trial and error, imperfection, nor ambiguity, in God's scientific creation, nor in His unfoldment of it.

Physics cannot truly be called a science if its antipode, metaphysics, is so identified. They are antagonistic one to the other. Physics is based solely on matter, and matter is illusion. It is without saying that distinguished physicists the world over have long suspected the substantiality of a material universe.

God's kingdom is a spiritual dominion, metaphysical in its every manifestation, and could not embrace so much as a grain of matter.

The famous physicist, Albert Einstein, learned in the

so-called logic of matter beyond virtually all men, has this to say about materiality and the real world of metaphysics:

"As always, the conception of the existence of the real world is fundamental in physics. Without it, there would be no borderline between psychology and physics. Those laws are always looked on as governing physical reality, and modern developments have changed nothing in this respect. The fact is we are today by no means sure about the conceptional basis of physics, and this state of uncertainty makes thoughtful physicists more conscious of the logical freedom in the choice of those concepts, as it was before the rise of quantum—and relativity theory, when the choice of the elementary concepts seemed beyond any doubt."

When such a profound thinker as Mr. Einstein, whose penetration into infinite space commands the respect of fellow scientists everywhere, is himself in doubt about the conceptional basis of physics—for indeed there can be no other basis for physics than that which is conceived—who is it that might be so presumptuous as to designate the phenomenon of matter a science?

To be sure, this noted physicist has not erred in so far as his cosmic calculations are concerned, but rather has he misapprehended—if he has—the nature of the substance out of which the cosmos is created. In fact, his inspiring explorations actually have been made into the realm of the metaphysical, or spiritual, universe, but his sense perception cognized its substance as a physical phenomenon. Notwithstanding this misinterpretation, he is obliged to concede none the less that metaphysical law is fundamental in governing what he assumes to be physical reality.

If the real world, as well as yourself, is not spiritual,

Mr. Einstein could never have misinterpreted the nature of creation in the first place, for the reason that there would be no Mr. Einstein existent to misinterpret. For even this greatly respected scientist is compelled to admit that creation must be interpreted through conceptional appreciation. Is this not what Jesus inferred, when he said:

"The kingdom of God is within you."?

Why then look for a material creation outside of yourself? Or for your own individuality in matter?

Perhaps what Mr. Einstein had not thoroughly grasped through his latent spiritual sense is this: the whole universe, with all its interstellar and spatial distances, resides in God's mind, and is therefore solely spiritual, or mental, as the characters, scenes and unfoldment in a stage presentation are the creations in the mind of the playwright conceiving it. Moreover, Mr. Einstein, with due respect for his wisdom and contributions to mankind, is the reflection, or image, of all that is in this mind of God's, not materially but spiritually.

This is the kingdom, which Jesus spoke of, that inherently is *in* Mr. Einstein; for were it not in him, he could never for an instant be aware of it. It is the selfsame kingdom which is in you, and me, and in the untutored rustic splitting rails in the backwoods country of the Ozarks. If creation is not purely a conscious manifestation, how then could it possibly be conceived by you and me?

Matter is simply an image of thought in the human mind, regardless of how much of it you perceive. Materiality does not, and cannot, exist anywhere else.

Among Gautama Buddha's last words, on his death-bed, concerning the illusion of material life, were these:

"All that is born, brought into being and put together, carries within itself the necessity of dissolution."

Matter could hardly be better defined than in this pithy observation that materialism is the seed of its own destruction.

Conversely, the philosophy that man and the cosmos are indestructible, perfect and eternal, was the basis of Jesus' teachings. If this were not so, how else could he have raised Lazarus, among others, from the grave, healed the hopelessly sick, stilled the turbulent waves, and assure all posterity, thus:

"He that believeth on me, the works that I do shall he do also; and greater works than these shall he do."?

Physics, in appraising an objective Nature existing independently of the Mind creating it, gives the lie to the soil wherein materialism takes root. Matter has neither substance nor genuine existence in its own right. Its constitution is wholly mental, and it exists merely as a false conception in the human mind.

Man knits his brow in a quandary over the Scriptures, tongue in cheek and plagued with doubt, when the clergy tells him with orthodoxical authority that the incidents in which Jesus walked on the water and fed the multitude were miracles.

In theology, a miracle is an event out of its established order, and possible only by divine intervention.

To explain away so great a lesson by interpreting these deeds as supernatural acts, exercised through a special dispensation of God, is to admit a lamentable lack of understanding as to its true import. If such explanations are designed to satisfy man's faculties for reasoning, this man in whom the kingdom of God resides, then the lesson which the Master had taught has been lost to all Christendom.

These marvels are no more miraculous in the eyes of one who understands the truth of being than is a problem in trigonometry to the mathematician. It is to the uninitiated that these performances are incomprehensible. This fact was recognized by the sage Goethe, who said:

"Things that are mysterious are not necessarily miracles."

If walking on the water and feeding the hungry multitude, as Jesus had demonstrated, are not perfectly natural acts rather than miraculous phenomena, why then did he tell us that we are equally capable of doing these same works, and even greater works than these?

It is utterly inconsistent to expect rational seekers after the truth to believe for an instant that a special dispensation of the Almighty was required to perform these works. The power to produce what appears to be miracles is *always* present when the truth is known, and profoundly felt, that man is not material, but spiritual consciousness alone.

For what other reason would the kingdom of God be within man, if not for the express purpose of performing these very works which Jesus had demonstrated?

That Jesus was no more in possession of the kingdom of God than you and I, Peter made clear:

"Of a truth I perceive that God is no respecter of persons."

The Master was no differently constituted than the rest of us, except of course that he understood, expressed and demonstrated the truth beyond all other men; and this truth is the fact that matter is nonexistent. He was primarily a teacher with deep spiritual insight, an oracle, but not God, nor a *special* son, as Peter had explicitly pointed out, any more than the other prophets and seers that breathe through the pages of Scripture.

Jesus was merely an exemplar of what he taught, proving by continual demonstration the capabilities of man, and inciting us to do likewise.

It is the time-honored deification of him with the investiture of a god, which the clergy has illogically inculcated in humankind through repeated admonition, that has separated us—farther than we wish to admit—from both this great teacher and his teachings.

The works which Jesus had made evident were not feats of legerdemain, effected for the purpose of overwhelming a gullible populace. God does not lend His power to beguile. Whatsoever God does, He gives His image the power to do likewise.

Indeed, it is the human appeal about Jesus that we love most, the humbling of himself in that he might raise us to his level of spiritual understanding, his patience in instructing those whom he taught, his confident assurance that we too can do the works which he had done, and greater wonders than these can we do.

If Jesus were truly God, as many are inclined to believe, or any of the ecclesiastical titles paralleling divine Providence, and such omnipotence is requisite to repeat his so-called miracles, how could you and I *possibly* emulate his mighty works, mortals that we supposedly are?

There is only *one* God, and He is the Creator. Jesus is *not* this One, nor is his identity in the Creator any different than is yours or mine. Jesus, and you and I, are specifically God's image, or the reflection of His conscious Self. This image is the kingdom and power of God that is within *all* of us, Jesus not excluded. It was the Master's penetrating insight into the truth of being, and its demonstration, rather than any ascendency to the Godhead, that has set him apart from his fellow men.

The humanity of Jesus has been placed by the clergy not only beyond the reach of us mortals, but beyond their own. It was the greatest of errors to disseminate this transcendent sanctification on so many generations of receptive thought. Had we been taught that Jesus was constituted as we are, no more nor less, save of course for his great spiritual power, we then would have looked with still greater wonder upon him in that he had overcome every physical obstacle. It would have been similar to our admiration for any preeminent personage whom most of us have the desire to emulate.

Had we been taught instead that the Nazarene was of the same clay as you and I, it would have been a challenge to the best in us to go and do likewise, because then we would know such emulation at least was possible of achievement. That this is so, Jesus reaffirmed; and the force of his exhortations still ring above the hue and cry of nearly two thousand years of ecclesiastical confusion.

But, no, we have been taught that he is God, or almost God; and then we are asked to do the very works that he has done. Obviously, this is inconsistent, since Jesus refuted any claim to the Godhead, thus:

"And the scribe said unto him, Master, thou hast said the truth: for there is one God; and there is *none other* but He . . . And when Jesus saw that he answered discreetly, he said unto the scribe, Thou art not far from the kingdom of God."

This passage in St. Mark clearly implies that there is no ambiguity of Trinity, Three in One, or One in Three; but rather is *everything* which He created *one* in Him.

Paul enlarges upon this point:

"The Spirit Itself beareth witness with our spirit, that we are the children of God: and if children, then heirs; heirs of God, and joint heirs with Christ."

If there still remains any question as to God's *oneness,* these words from the Master ring with a clarity that should dispel the final doubt:

"I ascend unto my Father, and *your* Father; and to my God, and *your* God."

Jesus made no distinction between himself and the rest of humanity. He never regarded himself by either word or deed as being superior in divine heritage to his fellow beings despite his higher understanding of the deific design. He had declared emphatically that we *all* are *one,* including himself, *in* God. It has rather been the founders of religious creeds that had taken upon themselves the authority to clothe this teacher of truth with the omnipotent character of God.

But far more humble than his overzealous canonizers, Jesus fortunately had made it clear that anyone was capable of doing the works that he had done. And, more, they could do even greater works, so he declared, than he had done.

Ralph Waldo Emerson, philosopher, clergyman and poet, touching upon this canonization, said:

"The position that men have given to Jesus, now for many centuries of history, is a position of authority. It characterizes only themselves. It cannot alter the eternal facts."

Incidentally, Jesus' ascension was not his material body rising into space. Such a belief is archaic and puerile. There is absolutely nothing material that could possibly ascend. God's mind is not a haven for material phenomena, nor is God separate from Jesus in that the latter had to rise to Him. It was rather in thought, or understanding, that he had risen. God is right where Jesus had stood. God is *always* wherever you and I and everybody else happens to be.

To accept literally that which plainly symbolizes an incomprehensible act is but to becloud its significance.

The fact of the ascension is this: Jesus completely overcame the final barrier of a material body through the ultimate realization of the truth of being. Spiritually aware, as he was, that matter was nonexistent, his supposedly physical body naturally disappeared into its native nothingness before the very eyes of those that beheld it materially. To be more specific, he merely rose above their physical sense understanding, the illusion of matter that still predominated their consciousness.

The Master had realized, consciously, the full import of spiritual reality. There never actually was a material body, not even among the eyewitnesses that believed they were looking out from one upon this seeming disappearance of another.

There is no other explanation of the ascension, unless it be one far-fetched and irrational.

If matter were real, such a visible ascent as Jesus was presumed to have made would be a self-evident impossibility, seeing that God is Spirit. Conversely, spiritual truth *does* make it possible for the very reason that matter is nothing more than a mistaken *belief* of substance.

Paul confirms this fact:

"Flesh and blood cannot inherit the kingdom of God."

Why not?

Simply because there is no matter existent, not so much as a pinch of it. Matter is merely a belief in human consciousness that spiritual reality is material. It is sheer absurdity, as Paul had plainly set forth, to believe the Master ascended to heaven in a material body, and sat on the right hand of God in flesh and blood.

Jesus was, and still is, the same image of God as you, and I, and the Brazilian fisherman pulling out an eel off the banks of the Amazon.

Our love and esteem for him is none the less profound merely because he is regarded as being of the same so-called clay as ourselves. The fact that this is so makes him rather a greater inspiration to follow.

Naturally our adoration, in its divine sense, can go out effectively only to God, and to God alone. The Master himself, throughout his entire ministry, instructed us explicitly to this end.

To be sure, we owe Jesus endless homage in that he has shown us the way to *truth* through precept and demonstration; but it was not he that inherently possessed the power to do the works of truth. The source of this authority is in divine Providence. This authority Jesus simply reflected, or expressed, as we all reflect and express in the degree that we understand its application. The true power belongs solely to God.

The Master made this very plain:

"I can of mine own self do nothing . . . for what things soever God doeth, these also doeth the Son likewise."

Is this not the image, or likeness, doing as its Creator does? John, too, clarifies this point:

"Behold, what manner of love the Father hath bestowed upon us, that we should be called the sons of God . . . *now* are we the sons of God."

Even the Psalmist was constrained to sing:

"Give unto the Lord the glory due unto His name."

Jesus was no more a preferred son of God than are you and I. Peter confirmed this fact when he said God is no respecter of persons. This is clearly seen when the truth of being is understood. There is only *one* Son, or Man, whom God created. This is the image of Himself. This man, held eternally intact in His mind, is wholly a conscious idea; and it is this idea whom you and I and Jesus, in this selfsame Consciousness, are the likeness or reflection. Moreover, you and I are as eternal as this idea which God sustains in His mind.

That this is so, John substantiates:

"The only begotten Son . . . is in the bosom of the Father."

The Son can never for an instant be outside of the Father. He is eternally *in* Him, in His consciousness. That Son, through image or reflection, is you and me, and the rustic hoeing a field of potatoes in Arkansas, no less than the great teacher of the Christian world.

Dr. Robert A. Millikan, noted physicist and Nobel prize winner, said:

"A purely materialistic philosophy is to me the height of unintelligence."

Dr. Millikan merely echoed the conviction uttered by the distinguished Bishop Berkeley nearly two hundred fifty years ago. There is *no* other way of explaining the so-called miracles which Jesus performed except by meta-physics, and metaphysics is absolutely spiritual.

To illustrate, let us examine the incident wherein the Master walked upon the wave-tossed sea, for this act proves beyond all question that the only substance there is abides in consciousness. This substance is thought. Nothing truly exists outside of consciousness, much less matter.

Those looking out from the ship, in the midst of the sea, thought they beheld a spirit moving across the water toward them. When, directly, the approaching Jesus spoke assuringly to the astounded onlookers, Peter beseeched the Master to call him thither so that he might likewise walk upon the waves. And being thus called, the disciple immediately came down from the ship and started to walk out on the billows to meet Jesus; but midway on the water he cried out for help, beginning suddenly to sink.

Jesus, stretching forth his hand, caught Peter up, and said:

"O thou of little faith, wherefore didst thou doubt?"

Peter, who obviously was not yet risen to the degree of spiritual faith necessary to completely overcome the belief that both he and the water were material, began to sink in what he still believed was fluid matter, inasmuch as the physical laws of matter precluded such an act.

But such was not the case with Jesus. The Master knew with solid conviction that he was spiritual idea alone, the image and likeness of God, and that the water similarly was spiritual idea. And, more, he was acutely aware that both these ideas were held eternally and securely in the mind that is God's, where neither matter nor mishap can possibly exist.

Had Peter's faith not been clouded with doubt that moment, he would have consummated to his glory this great demonstration. Physical law is simply a conscious but erroneous belief that substance is material.

There can be no accident nor catastrophe in God's mind; and there is *nothing* outside of His mind, despite all the seeming evidence of it to the contrary. God is One, the *only* Mind, and everything which He created is part and parcel of this one Mind. The only thing misadventure can possibly touch is the *belief* that any one of God's ideas is material. And such a belief is but a vision of illusory thought in the mind of a mortal.

Had Jesus believed he was constituted of matter, he would never have been able to walk on the waves, no more than Peter, nor could he have saved his disciple under *any* circumstances.

God does not suspend the majesty of His laws to prove something contrary to His own nature. Such a belief is absurd. Orthodoxy calls that which it does not understand a miracle, but this is because orthodoxy is unable to explain natural law and its unfoldment in any other way.

According to Genesis:

"On the seventh day God ended His work which He had made."

Surely this should signify that He was *finished* with His creation. Is it not then unreasonable to believe that God took up His work again merely to reverse some few operations of His law, after it already was declared:

"He saw every thing that He had made, and, behold, it was very good."?

It is evident that the people of Jesus' day lacked the faith to profitably assimilate the truth which he taught and demonstrated, for he said of them:

"They seeing see not; and hearing they hear not, neither do they understand. . . . For this people's heart is waxed gross, and their ears are dull of hearing, and their eyes they have closed."

The truth seemed to them so far beyond comprehension, as it does with mankind generally today, that they were disposed to believe Jesus more a deity than a human being like themselves. Yet we are told, by St. John:

"He that overcometh shall inherit all things."

Overcome what?

The illusion of matter of course.

Ask yourself, in the depths of your soul, what *else* is there to overcome?

Overcoming the illusion of matter was the supreme and final proof made by Jesus that materiality has no basis in fact. Were matter real, Jesus could never have healed the sick, transformed the sinner, and overcome death. All truth is embraced in spiritual consciousness, and is *never* in rapport with the belief in matter.

The philosopher, Jean Jacques Rousseau, said:

"All that comes from the Creator's hand is perfect, but when it falls into the hands of man it is spoilt."

Why is this so?

Simply because man inverts everything spiritual which he apprehends, and perceives it as material, thus he instantly spoils the true substance of God's idea. Mortal man mistakenly believes spiritual creation is material, and what obviously is mistaken in conception must by its erring nature be imperfect. Matter, in its most favorable light, is merely a disintegrating thought, originating not in God's mind, but in human consciousness alone.

When you have fairly overcome the belief that God has created His kingdom out of matter, you shall proportionally inherit *all* things, as promised by St. John. And only then will you clearly recognize, and consciously feel, the perfect and eternal man that you are, not materially but spiritually.

There is no other way of appreciating the kingdom of God within you than through the medium of your mentality. Your sense perception of its true substance is deceiving, as is the seeming movement of the sun in its relation to the earth. It is the mind that sees, hears, smells, tastes and feels, not any material organs.

Seeing the truth in this unerring perspective plausibly explains the episode of the loaves and the fishes. Notwithstanding that there were some five thousand hungered men, women and children assembled on the desert with only five loaves and two fishes, yet did Jesus pray to God for additional sustenance, which immediately was forthcoming, and all did eat of it. And when he was finished with teaching the five thousand, they took up twelve full baskets of what remained.

Indeed, there was nothing unnatural, or supernatural, about this noteworthy experience, nor did God suspend His laws temporarily so that this demonstration might be fulfilled.

The Master knew, and felt, with absolute certainty that all these five thousand hungered people were the express image of God, as he was, and that they existed spiritually in His mind. They could not possibly have any other existence. Asking his Father for that which they were in need obviously would be answered in the same spiritual substance of which he and they were made.

He put it very plain:

"Whatsoever ye shall ask in prayer, believing, ye shall receive."

Is it not reasonable then that a God of Spirit should rain down upon His children spiritual, rather than material, loaves and fishes, considering that these offspring were the spiritual image of Himself?

The great lesson to be learned, and impressed indelibly upon our consciousness, is this observation by Jesus:

"If ye then, being evil, know how to give good gifts unto your children, how much more shall your Father which is in heaven give good things to them that ask Him?"

The five thousand that ate of the spiritual sustenance perceived it materially, believing they were eating the substance of matter. This belief was merely an illusion, a material sense of the loaves and fishes. Jesus, on the other hand, saw the ineffable truth. He saw reality, the fact that they were feeding on spiritual sustenance alone, the entire performance being a manifestation of the mind. He knew that *all* was solely spiritual consciousness, and that there was nothing of matter that could possibly enter into this or any other demonstration of reality, even though it appeared so to the five thousand that ate of the nourishment.

Similarly explained is the mystery of the sycamine tree, plucked up by its root and planted into the sea by merely addressing it to do so. The tree, it must be seen, is a product exclusively of Mind, not of matter. Were the tree actually material, it would have been a self-evident impossibility to accomplish.

This interpretation accounts for the sun standing still for a whole day at the behest of Joshua. Were the sun really material, it could never possibly have been stayed in its course, even in its appearance of movement which we all know is an optical illusion. Too, this selfsame truth that *all* is Mind reveals as well the incident of the Red Sea, when the waters divided and the children of Israel passed through a corridor of the sea to the opposite side. Indeed, the material rod which Moses carried held no such power to divide the waters.

The power is in Mind, God; and this Mind is the kingdom which Jesus said is in you, and me, and the nomad wandering through the Gobi desert.

Herein lies the only rational answer to Jesus' amazing entrance through a door closed to outside admittance, yet appearing in the midst of his assembled disciples. Strange as this act seemed to the eleven startled men, it required no resort whatever to the magic arts. It was the conscious idea of spiritual man, in the image and likeness of God, passing through like substance. Had Jesus believed for a fleeting instant that he or the door, or both, was material, he could never have gained entrance.

All the so-called miracles recorded in the Scriptures, the numerous healings and inexplicable acts performed by Jesus, Daniel walking unharmed in the lions' den, and Shadrach, Meshach and Abednego in the midst of the fiery furnace, are similarly accounted for, that man is not material, but spiritual.

The Master's ascension, beyond all material perception, was a complete and perfect realization of this divine consciousness.

Matter is nothing more than the mist of thought.

CHAPTER V

Does all this seem incredible to you, that matter is merely an illusion and that we and everything about us are solely conscious ideas in God's mind?

If so, what then must be your reaction to *this* remarkable assurance given us by the Master:

"If ye have faith as a grain of mustard seed, ye shall say unto this mountain, remove hence to yonder place; and it shall remove; and nothing shall be impossible to you."?

Think of it! *Nothing* shall be impossible to you.

Do you believe him? You, a devout adherent of his teachings?

How else, but by mentally resolving the illusion of matter into its true counterpart, whose reality is *idea* alone, spiritualized thought, could this mountain be removed?

Only mortal man, who believes himself to be material but definitely is not, sees everything as matter.

All the substance there is to you and me, to a blade of grass, a soaring eagle, or the constellation Andromeda, is the consciousness which comprises God's innumerable ideas, and these ideas are all that have actual existence. They can abide in no other place than in God's mind.

These ideas, including you and me, and the seasonal harvests that come up out of the ground, have all the spiritual qualities—symmetry, beauty, characteristics, color and growth—which you seem to see only as being material. But this is an illusion of a physical sense of things. You see, hear, feel, smell and taste your own thoughts, for it is in your mind alone that you experience what appears external to it.

Professor Samuel Pierpont Langley, physicist, astronomer, and inventor of the first aeroplane, said:

"The color of the rose is in ourselves."

In fact the entire rose is in ourselves, its substance, beauty, scent and color. Virtually all physicists today are agreed that color is indicated in the material world solely by diverse wave lengths registered on the color spectrum in ourselves. Of course this scientific consensus, although an honest endeavor in the right direction, is none the less a confused attempt to unite an illusory material world with ourselves.

There absolutely can be no material world outside of ourselves, anywhere. However, there most certainly *is* a spiritual world *in* us, our consciousness. This is God's creation, the kingdom which Jesus said is *within* us. There is no other creation, world, universe nor cosmos. Physical scientists still are struggling in the dark to harmonize the impossible, Spirit and matter, the truth and error. They see gleams of the truth occasionally, and these evidences of reality are unsatisfactorily fitted in with the predominant illusion.

Not only is the color spectrum in ourselves, as Professor Langley has pointed out, but the very objects themselves in which we see the color. When it is thoroughly seen that matter is nothing more than an unreal appearance of its

spiritual counterpart in your consciousness, then will the
Master's teachings begin to take on meaning and unfold
for you with a clarity of understanding that you had never
before thought possible.

Sir Arthur Stanley Eddington, world-renowned scientist
and professor of astronomy, perhaps has seen greater and
more convincing gleams of this truth than most of his fellow savants. He said:

> **"There is no color in the physical world. . . . The sensory
> qualities of color, sound and scent cannot be transmitted
> to us from the object in the external world to which we
> attribute the color, sound and scent."**

If there is no color in the physical world, as Professor
Eddington has stated, then there is *nothing* physical nor
material in this so-called world of matter. What you actually see is the spiritual world, the kingdom that is wholly
within you through conscious reflection, and this you in-
accurately perceive *outside* of yourself and then call it
matter.

To weigh this important point in still another light,
Bertrand Russell, distinguished philosopher and protag-
onist of the new mathematical logic, states in his Analysis
of Matter:

> **"What the physiologist sees when he examines a brain is in
> the physiologist, not in the brain he is examining."**

Why is this so?

If color, sound and scent, together with all the objects
from whence they originate, are in the physiologist, as
they are in you and me, so then must the inanimate brain
which he examines be in him also. Either *all* is in you, as

Jesus said it is, or not the least part of the kingdom is within you. There is no happy medium. Moreover, *all* is solely mental. There is nothing else, much less matter.

To further quote Sir James Hopwood Jeans:

"All earlier systems of physics, from the Newtonian mechanics down to the old quantum theory, fell into the error of identifying appearance with reality . . . without even being conscious of a deeper reality beyond. The new quantum theory has shown that we must probe the deeper substratum of reality before we can understand the world of appearance."

When this deeper substratum is ultimately probed by the physicists, as it surely will be in the not too distant future, it will then be learned that the material world of appearance is simply a deceptive picture in human consciousness.

Matter is *ever* illusion; and illusion always is the reverse of truth. To ascertain the truth of anything, you simply reverse what appears to be material into a conscious idea, its spiritual counterpart, in your thought, and this is all that is real of the thing reversed, including yourself. What appears to you as being physical is only an image of deceptive thought focussed on your mind.

Seeing yourself and everything in the universe as spiritual ideas in God's mind, the whole combining to make His *oneness,* or kingdom, enhances the reality of your true individuality at once, and gives a far clearer and more substantial awareness to existence.

You are the image of God as the motion picture on the screen is the image of the film unwinding in the projection room. You cannot exist without being sustained by

God any more than the moving images on the screen can be sustained without the unwinding film in the projection room.

Such is your coexistence with God. It is an indissoluble affinity.

You being the image of God is somewhat the same as your likeness in the mirror is the image of you. Were you wholly unaware that the mirror existed for the express purpose of reflecting your likeness, the reflection manifestly would be regarded by you as convincing evidence of the reality of matter. So it is that you identify yourself materially as the image, or reflection, of God.

To cite Sir Arthur Stanley Eddington again:

"Most of our common impressions of substance . . . have turned out to be illusory, and the externality of the world might be equally untrustworthy."

Now that we have God fairly established as universal Consciousness, and man a *conscious* image of Him, let us consider briefly His creation. It is only by visualizing the vastness and complexity of His infinite kingdom that we can begin to realize how glorious and beyond mortal man's limited comprehension is this exalted conception of the Most High.

Not only are the cosmos and its activities, and everything that evolves, has being, and breathes upon the innumerable planets, each with its peculiar destiny, held in perfect and eternal relation to every other idea in God's mind—for indeed God *is* MIND—but the very health, welfare and individual needs of the minutest idea dwells intact therein, and is ever tenderly cared for by its merciful Creator.

The Master said:

"The very hairs of your head are all numbered."

It is plain, from this disclosure, that man has nothing to fear upon this earth. God has foreseen his every need. All his anxieties are as unfounded and unreal as his belief that he is a material entity. Divine Wisdom sustains *everything* It has made, eternally and mercifully.

It would take a seeming eternity to enumerate the constituent elements and cohesions which establish God's ideas, and the multitudinous functions and responses that go on in each one, the revolutions of the countless luminaries in celestial space, the influences which one solar combination has on another, the tides and the seasons, and the general metamorphosis that ceaselessly goes on within the bowels of the revolving spheres to supply us with coal, and oil, and iron, and marble, and even diamonds to plight milady's affections.

Indeed, it is enough that we gape in wonder on the blue of the sky, the unerring laws of gravitation, the beauty and fragrance of a budding lilac bush, the song of a lark, golden wheat rippling in the breeze, two lovers gazing wistfully into a full moon. It is all spiritual, mental, knowing. None of it is material.

All of this, and that which still is beyond your remotest conception of what infinity implies, is yours.

Think for a brief moment what that means! *Yours!* All of it. To possess as your own. To appreciate. Utilize. Enjoy.

This is the kingdom of God that is within you.

And here you are, struggling and contending with one another for still more, breaking your back, and your spirit, and your very health, scheming and conniving and stealing to acquire more than your fellow man, when all the while the windows of heaven are everlastingly pouring down more than you can possibly use.

And for what purpose are you doing this?

Obviously, to gratify a mistaken belief that the greater your possession of this illusion of material riches, the more assured will be your present and future security, as if God already has not supplied every single one of us with the only genuine wealth existent. And so abundantly of it in fact that it is beyond the understanding of mortal man to conceive even of the smallest part.

Mortals try so desperately to seek security where it is impossible to be found. There is no such thing as, nor assurance of, material security, but merely an illusion of it is all.

Of material riches, Jesus said:

"Lay not up for yourselves treasures upon earth, where moth and rust doth corrupt . . . but lay up for yourselves treasures in heaven, where neither moth nor rust doth corrupt; for where your treasure is, there will your heart be also."

Only by laying up spiritual treasures can you establish *real* security. Such treasures are divinely correlated with the kingdom of God that is within you; and they bear far greater, more enduring, and infinitely better, fruit than is to be found in the illusion of material riches.

Yet, how many actually believe this?

This kingdom, which Jesus spoke of, eternally is unfolding new ideas, realities, for you to discover and utilize, like the internal combustion engine, radio, television, dress de-

signing, architecture, plastics and synthetics, a new principle for a washing machine, the progressive use of energy
—all to be brought forth and evolved in *mind,* never in
matter. All the forces and dynamics and continuities about
us are God's ideas, to be eventually discovered, adapted
and made practical use of, solely in our consciousness, and
must necessarily be sustained by a divine Creator. They
do not come into being from nothing.

Man perverts these ideas the instant he perceives and
acknowledges them materially. Such perversion obviously
brings in its wake all the disease, disorder and futility that
we daily experience.

Conversely, the glory of God truly is within you. He
stretches forth His arms, and literally speaks out:

"Son, what is Mine is thine; take full possession of it!"

Son! Think of the nobility that is yours! The son of
God! What a supreme privilege to be spiritually endowed
with this gift of kinship in the Almighty!

You are virtually the whole province of creation, a conscious facsimile of it to be exact, considering that God's entire and indivisible kingdom is within you. From the very
instant that you were cast in the matrix of spirituality,
you have been made a copartner in His dominion. To but
pause for a single moment and realize what this birthright
means, to consider its magnitude and grandeur, is to repeat what John was constrained to exclaim:

**"Behold, what manner of love the Father hath bestowed
upon us, that we should be called the sons of God!"**

Seeing that we are created solely in consciousness, we
can have but one medium of appreciation, and that is

realization, realizing the ideas of God which are—like our-selves—made out of the spiritual substance of His con-sciousness. If you are disposed to believe that there is any-thing else but consciousness to you, a tree, or the idling motor in your automobile, then you definitely are living in a world of illusion not far removed from the common dream. For such a belief subsists on the same train of thought that feeds both the illusion and the dream which you have in sleep.

Man is not *actually* a separate entity from the things which he observes. The irrefutable fact is that everything man observes, hears and feels, is within himself. This is the great departure from the belief that you and the uni-verse are material. It is the truth of being as revealed by Jesus, when he declared:

"The kingdom of God is within you."

Mind is not in body, but rather is body in mind. When you begin to see the light of this truth with reasonable clarity, you will begin to take proportional mastery over what appears to be your material body, and consequently bring to it sound health where disease, or the fear of it, prevailed.

Not only is your body in mind, but the room in which you are reading this volume is in mind. Yes, *your* so-called mind which you believe is in your body. Indeed, you are not in the room—that is to say your physical body is not in a room constructed of matter—despite all your protests to the contrary. The room specifically is *in* you.

Think not that this is incredible. It is the absolute *truth*. The very substance and power of God's creation is the consciousness constituting His universal idea. There never was nor ever will be matter. It is merely illusion, notwith-standing its hard appearance and solid feel in the grasp of your hand. You must reverse the unreal material appear-ance, of both yourself and the physical aspects of the room, if you would arrive at the spiritual reality. And there can be *no* other reality.

Is it not obvious that you must be conscious of the room to recognize it? If this is so, then the room must definitely be *in* your consciousness. Not outside of it. It can *never* exist outside the pale of consciousness. If the kingdom of God is within you, surely so infinitesimal a part of it as the room you are sitting in could hardly be excluded. Nothing can be outside of you, whether it be your body, the room, or the neighbor across the street.

Had Jesus not been aware of this revealing truth, he could never have healed the legion of sick by the mere ex-pedient of thought, particularly those that were far remote from his proximity. He knew that *everybody* and *every-thing* were within him through conscious reflection, and therefore *all* that God had made was within his immediate presence, notwithstanding the material concept of spatial distance.

The important point concerning you and the room is this: the room, you will agree, cannot think to include you; but, on the contrary, you do the thinking and conse-quently include the room within *your* consciousness. Mind gives abode only to that which is mental. It would be utterly impossible for mind to harbor within itself, or to recognize outside of itself, so much as a grain of material substance. It knows of no such thing as actual matter; nor can mind see, hear, feel, smell or taste matter, inasmuch as it is a purely mental domain. Mind, however, conceives and experiences a *sense* of matter, a mere picture of it is all, projected in color and third dimension upon the mirror of consciousness.

What mind really sees, hears, feels, smells and tastes, is its own thoughts. It can see, hear, feel, smell and taste *nothing* outside of itself. This is obvious, since nothing exists outside of consciousness. It is well here to impress deeply upon your faculties of awareness the fact that mind is not in a material body, but rather is this illusion of a material body, with all its density, viscera and activity, in mind. And it is in this selfsame mind that the room also has its presence, or existence, seeing that it was constructed mentally in the first place, and with *mental* building materials, ideas.

To draw out the illustration further: if a corpse were placed in this controversial room, the corpse apparently would have no more knowledge of being in the room than the room would be aware that the corpse was within its four walls. Yet, within this deceased body are a brain that cannot think, eyes that cannot see, ears that cannot hear, hands that cannot feel, a nose that cannot smell, and a tongue that cannot taste.

The question arises: what then is it that knows or perceives?

Inasmuch as neither the room nor the corpse is conscious of each other, or of anything in fact, both evidently must be material illusions in the presence of the mind *entertaining* them. They can have no other existence than in this mind. Moreover, this latter picture clearly sets forth the manner in which man imprisons himself, and frequently to his own detriment, within his erring thoughts.

Should you tell yourself that the life which departed

from the corpse naturally left it impotent to think and act, you unwittingly will strengthen the logic of truth's unfoldment.

What is life if it is not consciousness? Have you ever observed one without the other?

The truth about the corpse is this: life had never departed from it, but rather had the erroneous *belief* of a material body departed from the carnal mind entertaining this illusion of a body. Life *never* was in the corpse, nor is it ever in *any* material body, even when it appears so. It is utterly impossible for life to be in a material body inasmuch as there is no matter existent. The corpse is simply the decomposition of material *belief,* the last stage of an illogical conviction that once assumed it possessed life.

Can God's image and likeness disintegrate?

Hardly.

The only thing that can know existence, to have knowledge of God's creation, is that which is conceived in His consciousness alone. That is all. Whatever is conceived in God's consciousness must necessarily exist *in* It eternally and in its pristine perfection. Such consciousness knows nothing outside of itself. It absolutely has no cognizance of matter, even though matter were existent, which it is not. What appears to be material is but a counterfeit, in belief only, of spiritual reality.

This explains why your awareness of things is confined solely to thought; for without consciousness to objectify these thoughts, or things, in your mind, there could be nothing to be aware of, or to realize. Both a material room and a material body, if they were possible of existence outside of yourself—which of course is contrary to truth—

could never under *any* circumstance be cognized by consciousness. This is so because consciousness sees, knows, actuates and appreciates only such evidences of awareness as are within itself.

That which you see as your physical body is merely a three-dimensional outline of false belief in the lens of your supposed mind, the selfsame mind which you assume is *within* this illusory body. Not only the room under discussion, but the house you live in, is in your mind, as are the earth and universe. Your whole existence, environment, ambitions, loves and hates and fears—yes, all you conceive is within you, within your mind. You merely project it outside of yourself in thought.

When you see a tree in your thought outside of yourself, you see it materially as something which appears impossible to bring inside of this thought again, because you fancy yourself material too.

Always keep in mind this verity: ideas are things; or, conversely, things are ideas, and exist only in your mind by reflection. These ideas, thus mentally visible to your consciousness, are the only language whereby God informs and impresses you with His creation and its varied activities.

Nothing actually is conceived by you from without, seeing that there is *nothing* outside of you. Everything you conceive already is within you, and you externalize it *without* solely in your consciousness, in thought, not matter.

This divine panorama of true being that seems so concretely outside of yourself is the kingdom of God that is *within* you.

CHAPTER VI

DOES THIS philosophy of true being seem to you somewhat far-fetched to reasonably accept?

None the less, this is the kingdom that God had created, and which Jesus said is wholly within you.

Ask yourself, humbly:

"How else but by mental reflection, through the medium of mind, can this kingdom be within me?"

The answer is self-evident on the basis of reason alone. It is an incontrovertible fact whether you wish to recognize its logic or not. You cannot possibly escape it. It is what you are. It is what God ordained. It is His essence, design and enterprise. It is the only *being* existent, and such being resides solely in consciousness. It is the kingdom we *all* reflect, consciously.

The question resolves itself to this: do you wish to discover in yourself the purpose and substance of this priceless heritage? To better understand it? To more fully utilize it to the advantage for which it was created?

Or are you rather disposed to accept the confusion of material illusion, with all its discords, adversities, diseases, anxieties, ordeals and sorrows, none of which God is aware?

This kingdom, which Jesus spoke of, is in one respect similar to the multiplication table. If you are loath to recognize the principle of multiplication because you believe it untrue, and therefore ineffectual, you obviously will profit nothing from its use.

To understand what multiplication teaches, you first must inquire into its nature, and then apply it to the advantage for which it was created. Like the *one* perfect kingdom of God, there is but *one* perfect multiplication table, and it inherently is within every one of us to express in all its perfection. An imperfect solution, whatever it may be, has nothing in common with the correct one.

By the same token, if you are not at least vaguely aware that the kingdom of God is within you, then you are in the same darkness that one must be in about the multiplication table when he knows nothing at all of its purpose and application.

Such lack of insight into the truth of being is not unlike Plato's famous allegory.

The Greek philosopher portrayed mankind chained in a cave in such way that it could see only that which was reflected in shadow on the back wall. The busy life and activity of reality which went on outside the cave was not perceptible to mankind chained within, save by its shadows reflected by the sunlight on the back wall. In so far as mankind, chained within the cave, was concerned, these shadows constituted its only world of appearance, or phenomena; while the reality of the busy world outside the cave was ever beyond its cognizance.

So it is in actual existence. The reality of all things is equally beyond the cognizance of a humanity that sees no deeper into the truth of being than the mere appearance of material illusion. This state of misconception perceives little more than Plato's shadows on the wall.

Indeed, God did not sit at an immense work-bench with illimitable piles of matter at His fingertips out of which to create the planets and firmament, including yourself. Nor did He speak the immemorial *Word* and substance matter ensued. He created His kingdom in His mind. The finished creation exists nowhere else. God's ideas, unlike your own, are real and substantial, and endure throughout all eternity *in* His mind. There is *no* other creation nor kingdom. Whatever appears external to this Mind, in either thought or matter, is merely human invention or illusion.

If the author of a novel can create in his mind a tense and vivid drama in which the reader loses himself for a spell, wherein its several characters exchange stimulating conversation, perceive and appraise each other's designs and motives, travel considerable distances, and become influenced by the impelling emotions that have been affected, why then should the greater and far more interesting spectacle of the creation, with its innumerable characters and complex activities, conceived and sustained by God in *His* mind, be less credible to the same reader?

William Shakespeare, immortal bard, well said:

"All the world is a stage, and we are the actors."

The stage of this *real life* drama is the mind of God, the Author; and we, His actors, are merely repeating the lines of His infinite creation unfolding before our conscious receptivity.

Little wonder that Johannes Kepler was constrained to exclaim:

"O Lord, I am thinking Thy thoughts after Thee!"

We objectify our thoughts materially in consciousness, and enjoy or abhor their activities which we ourselves construct and empower, as surely as we project upon the tapestry of our minds the novel that we read. The unfoldment of the novel, as perceived in the reader's mind, is thought being made evident. None of it is material, nor is it enacted in material form, but in consciousness. Similarly is the reality of creation unfolded, in *your* consciousness, seeing that it was God's purpose to design it so.

Perhaps no more revealing picture of matter can be had than that set forth by J. W. N. Sullivan in the London *Observer,* reviewing Sir Arthur Stanley Eddington's contribution to the book, *Science, Religion and Reality.* Mr. Sullivan, himself an author of note in the physical sciences, said:

"According to Eddington, the science of physics, which is the basic science, is concerned only with the *form* of phenomena and not with their content. Of the intrinsic nature of matter science knows nothing, and never can know anything. Physics knows only paradoxical conclusions gained from readings on measuring instruments, and their relations to each other. As to what matter really *is,* the science of physics can tell us nothing. The laws of Nature are the results of the mind's own actions, and not something imposed on an independently existing universe from without. Indeed, not only the laws of Nature, but space and time and the material universe itself, are constructions of the human mind. The mind has not constructed all this out of nothing. The ultimate reality is structure, and from this fact the universe we know is deduced. Thus the existence of the universe becomes primarily a psychological problem. There is no reason in the nature of things why we should not know the future and have to deduce the past. To an altogether unsuspected extent the universe we live in is a creation of our own minds. The nature of it is forever outside of physical scientific investigation. Matter itself is mental."

As for knowing the future and deducing the past, Jesus similarly made allusion to this singular verity, thus:

"Ye can discern the face of the sky; but can ye not discern the signs of the times?"

Physics knows absolutely nothing of matter's content, other than that it is wholly mental phenomena. The famous physicist, Sir Arthur Stanley Eddington, who had given a lifetime of research to this moot subject, dared to lift his vision beyond present day conjecture. He said, moreover:

"Space and time are only approximate *conceptions*. . . . Like the systems of Euclid, of Ptolemy, of Newton, which have served their turn, so the systems of Einstein and Heisenberg may give way to some fuller realization of the world."

Such reasoning is progression. To hold stubbornly to antiquated theories and practices, whether they be scientific, religious or philosophic, is retrogression. Man can never hope to reach the spiritual heights of perfection so long as he believes himself to be constituted of, and sustained by, matter. Material knowledge is sheer deception. It has no basis in fact. It is a fallacy.

Of corporeal knowledge, the venerable Socrates said:

"As for me, all I know is that I know nothing."

This seems incredible, coming from one of such profound learning; but the fact remains that material knowledge from its very nature is *nothing,* seeing that matter does not exist, and anything akin to it must necessarily be without substance or being.

But this is not so of spiritual truth, in which all reality and divine intelligence are anchored.

Far more discerning than the Athenian philosopher was the famous English physicist, who saw the light of truth after lifelong research revealed the cosmos, space and time, within the mind of man himself.

Did not Jesus say the same thing:

"The kingdom of God is within you."?

What other interpretation could there possibly be of this kingdom within you than the fact that it is the creation itself, and the assurance that you have absolute

"dominion over every thing that moveth upon the earth."?

This amazing revelation which Jesus made known to all posterity is not some abstract theory put forward for the purpose of befuddling our thinking. On the contrary, it is the sublime *truth.*

His foremost object as a teacher was to arouse our dormant understanding so that we might avail ourselves profitably of this glorious possession within us. Strip away that part of the Biblical record dealing with his healing of bodily disease and infirmity—which he particularly stressed that you too are qualified to do, and even more than he had done can you do—and you strip away the spiritual character and purpose of his mission. Indeed, you strip away the Master's individuality itself.

What else than his demonstrations of healing has secured for him the perpetuation of his teachings?

The truth has too long been couched in cryptic approaches, in parables dressed in metaphor and trope, in theological dogma, and in the ignorance of material hypothesis. Let us rather put it on the table where it can be seen in clear view, in its undisguised state, and then examine it, probe into its nature, analyze it, experiment with it, and take full advantage of it as God intended we should.

Truth can be interpreted only spiritually. The best that physical science can hope to achieve in its researches is to lead us to the *illusion* of reality; and in this way the entire masquerade of matter, in all its forms of error, must inevitably be exposed.

Notwithstanding the fact that Jesus' teachings, and demonstrations thereof, have provoked so many generations of Christians to revere his name, comparatively few fairly understood and practiced the pith of what he taught.

The Master declared:

"I am come that they might have life, and that they might have it more abundantly."

To be sure, he was not alluding to the materialism which is so rampant in life today, what with its periods of prosperity and want, amassing of riches by the few, universal poverty, exalted belief of being a superior being or race, the common evils of malice, hatred, intolerance, and a host of similar errors rising out of materialistic confusion.

Rather was the Galilean teacher alluding to life as spiritual, and *not* material, and man the son of God, whom the Father adequately cares for at *all* times. He knew only too well that it was through such realization, in consciousness, that man can possibly come into this more abundant life. He knew that in no other way, but spiritually, will man

"love God with all his heart . . . and his neighbor as himself."

This spiritual man in the image of God, and there can be no other man, need *never* be crushed in health and spirit between the grinding wheels of materialism for the mere privilege of eking out a bare subsistence. If you are disposed to believe that this abundant life, which Jesus spoke of, is material, then you are simply pursuing an existence that *appears* otherwise than what it really is.

Consider soundly: for what else could this promise of an abundant life imply, than freeing yourself from the material illusion that has bound you to disease, pain, evil, want, discontent, and the whole gamut of its corrupt relationship?

It should be obvious that God did not make these errors. Everything that He had made, we are told, was *good*.

Indeed, these evils are false beliefs which *you* alone have externalized in your own thought, and then see in all their ugliness as material. These are the gods that you worship, believing as you do that such mental aberrations are realities, when the truth is they are only illusions, in your consciousness.

Actually there is *no* evil, other than that which man himself conceives and objectifies in his own consciousness. Certainly God did not create it.

Habakkuk, the prophet, said of God:

"Thou art of purer eyes than to behold evil, and canst not look on iniquity."

Your own evil thoughts, which you yourself have evolved, are the seed of all your fears. There is absolutely nothing else that you *can* fear, since nothing can possibly exist outside of your consciousness. Thus you build a Frankenstein which in the end inevitably consumes the very illusion which you mistakenly believe is your true self. Such belief is as fictitious as is the terrifying tale of Shelley's monster, and no less destructive to your well-being.

Fear, in whatever light you look at it, is but the illusion of something nonexistent. If you are made in God's image, and sustained by Him, your fear of *anything* is as groundless as your belief that you are material.

Fear and evil are destroyed, as are all errors, through the realization that you are the spiritual child of God, and reside as *one* eternally with Him in His mind, and *not* in matter.

To define man from another point of view, he is God's understanding of Himself, and this understanding is purely a mental picture, or conscious reflection. The more you learn to know God under these circumstances, the more perfect you will become and proportionally know yourself. It is by constantly endeavoring to identify yourself with Him that you attune yourself with true being. Only by recognizing existence as solely spiritual can you discover your real identification.

In Psalms, we are told:

"He that dwelleth in the secret place of the Most High shall abide under the shadow of the Almighty."

What a refreshing thought is this divine privilege of abiding under the shadow of God, wherein you are secure in His health, abundance and eternal protection! Not materially is this so, but spiritually. You need only to *think* these forces into the activities of your daily experience. It is obvious that matter cannot dwell in the secret place of the Most High. This prerogative is reserved for spiritual consciousness alone, the substance out of which man is made. This consciousness not only receives the reward, but *is* the reward.

Jesus made this clear, when he said:

"It is the Spirit that quickeneth; the flesh profiteth *nothing.*"

We are the sons of God in the degree that we reflect Him, spiritually, in His image and likeness; and this reflection is entirely mental. To be sure, we are not separate entities in the sense that each one of us contains in himself an independent existence, unsustained and ungoverned by the Creator of all things. Such a state of being is unthinkable. You could no more have existence as a separate entity than one of your own ideas, conceived in your mind, could have a separate existence from you.

Man is subordinate to God. He lives *in* his Creator. In God's mind. Were the Almighty to withdraw that which He reflects as His image, man and all the creation would that instant disappear into nothingness, as your own idea would similarly disappear if you were to dissociate it from your thought. Everything lives in thought; matter merely usurps it, as an unreal belief.

The Psalmist declared:

"The fool hath said in his heart, There is no God."

Let us further illustrate what man is as God's image, so that a more vivid picture may be had of this wondrous conception which you are.

Assume that you are standing before a number of mirrors placed at varying angles, each returning and thereby greatly multiplying your image into each of the other mirrors. Obviously you would see yourself reflected countless times, and yet be certain in your own mind that there is but *one* you. So it is with man in God's likeness, or reflection.

There is in reality but one Son, one Man, one Body, and that one is what God sees of Himself. This conscious knowledge which He has of His *oneness* is reflected to your human sense as an infinity of sons, men, or bodies, as is the multiplied reflection of your mortal self in the mirrors. The dawning of this light in your consciousness is spiritual awareness.

This awareness is what is meant as man made in the image of God.

Your individuality is simply *realizing* what God sees of Himself, for such is His image, the only substance there is to your identity. This realization is the actual image which you are, not in matter but in mind. The clearer that you learn to see this truth, the more distinct will become the outline of your own individuality in this selfsame consciousness.

There is no other way nor place in which you can have existence.

Paul put it even more to the point:

"They which are the children of the flesh, these are *not* the children of God."

Of course not! God's children are formed of the substance of His mentality, or Spirit. They were *never* cast in matter. It is self-evident that the children of the flesh *must* be illusion if they are not the children of God.

This one perfect Man, or Son, which God holds forever intact in His mind is you, and me, and Chung Lee in the hinterlands of China, John Burke who lives in the moors of England, and the shopkeeper Nehrdu on the Ganges in India. He is every human being of the white, black, red, brown and yellow races; and here it is well to mention the fact that superiority of race is as much illusion, or fable, as is the belief that humankind lives in matter.

The kingdom of God is in every one of the foregoing individuals in the degree that he understands, and puts into practice, the truth of being. Indeed he *is* the truth in eternal manifestation.

Paul, clarifying this individuality of man as the image of God, exposes the very inanity of nationalism and bigotry, thus:

"There is neither Jew nor Gentile, there is neither bond nor free, there is neither male nor female. . . . All are baptised into *one* body. . . . All have been made to drink into *one* Spirit."

This significant disclosure by the apostle brings into sharp focus man's ignorance of true being, as well as the darkness out of which he forges his material concepts.

Paul further amplified:

"If any man think that he knoweth any thing, he knoweth nothing yet as he ought to know."

Mortal man's knowledge for the most part is academic and based wholly on matter. As a consequence, the materialism of the ages growing out of this fallacious belief has erroneously molded the thinking of all mankind.

John Fiske, noted scientist and philosopher, expressly pointed out this error of mortal thinking:

"It was long ago shown that all the qualities of matter are what the mind makes them, and have no existence as such, apart from the mind."

From time immemorial men of profound wisdom have questioned the common belief that man and the universe are the phenomena of matter. Another of these eminent sages, the philosopher and thinker, Immanuel Kant, declared:

"The world's life is only an appearance, a sensuous image of the pure spiritual life . . . a dream, and having no reality in itself."

You are the reflection of God's consciousness, and this mental image of Him is absolutely *all* there is to you. This is the truth about you, whether you wish to accept this status of your individuality or not. If you did not reflect God's consciousness there would be nothing to indicate your identity, for you would have none. You would be unconceived, a nonentity, nothing.

Notwithstanding its physical complexion, matter is an out-and-out illusion, an erroneous belief, and nonexistent. It has no more substance than a mirage. Any attempt to explain the composition of matter would be as ridiculous as analyzing the constitution of nothing. Seeing or feeling matter is merely seeing or feeling an inverted image in your mind.

Of this inversion, Isaiah said:

"Your turning of things upside down shall be esteemed as the potter's clay: for shall the work say of Him that made it, He made me not?"

Your physical *sense* of things tells you that you are material, and therefore substantial; and that which you sense as consciousness appears to you to be ethereal, or some immaterial emanation whose source supposedly is *in* matter. But it is the contrary that is true: for that which appears to your *sense* of the physical to be real is, in fact, unsubstantial; and that which you recognize as consciousness, and which seems ethereal, actually is the only true substance of which you are constituted.

It is out of this latter substance, divine consciousness, that you are made. Indeed, this does not infer that you are merely a shadowy outline in thought. The various elements, dimensions, quantities and densities that combine to constitute you, your heart and lungs and liver and stomach, together with all their activities, including the blood that flows through your veins, are vividly real; yet not so much as a jot of it is material. *All* of it is spiritual consciousness, the image which you are of God.

No less an integral part of this image are the inherent qualities of love and kindness, your intelligence, strength, abundance, happiness and initiative, among other things.

God sustains you in everything that you require for a contented and well-ordered life. No person, thing, nor circumstance, can deprive you of a single need or talent which your Father in heaven has given you, seeing that His entire kingdom is eternally within you.

Like the Psalmist, you, too, can sing out:

"The lines are fallen unto me in pleasant places; yea, I have a goodly heritage."

God never made an Irishman, a German, nor a Spaniard; neither did He make a Chinaman, an Indian, nor an Eskimo. The peculiar physical and linguistical characteristics of nationals, races and tribes are man-made. They are part and parcel of the illusion that God had cast man and the universe out of matter. Even such material knowledge as anatomy, anthropology and physiognomy are without spiritual basis; for, like the characteristics of different peoples, they express only the change and structural beliefs of mortal thought through the ages. And so it is with ethnology, genealogy, heredity, and other such phenomena of the human mind.

Man is, and always shall be, a slave to his own beliefs whenever these beliefs are based on the assumption that he is a physical structure rather than a conscious idea.

Inasmuch as we have fairly established the fact that the intrinsic nature of God, and man, and the creation, is purely spiritual consciousness, including no other substance, let us briefly consider here the Christ, and the part *it* plays in the divine order.

The truth, as unfolded by God before your consciousness, is the Christ. It is the evidence of creation. To enlarge upon this simple revelation with unintelligible hierarchic interpretations is to make obscure that which is obviously comprehensible.

The Christ is merely the kingdom of God, and all that this kingdom implies, dawning with increasing clarity upon your understanding. It is the truth acquainting you not only with the source of all life and supply, but with their ever availability and enjoyment. Specifically, the Christ is your conscious realization of the presence of God, and the communication of His creation to you.

Availing yourself of the kingdom of God in your life is evidencing, in the ratio to your understanding, the illimitable Christ, or ideal man.

Jesus was a perfect example of this manifestation, expressing the full power of truth. We *all*, to a smaller extent, manifest the Christ in our individual endeavors to attune ourselves more perfectly with God. Jesus' greater understanding of the truth, that all reality is in Spirit and Its unfoldment through consciousness, naturally lifted him into a higher degree of harmony with the Christ.

Experiencing this harmony, or understanding of the Christ, is having unity with God. This state of divine realization is no less possible for you to attain than it was for Jesus. Such awareness of the deific design is the *only* reality there is. The Master made it plain throughout all his teachings that this perfect state of being is *within* every one of us. It needs merely to be evidenced.

The Christ is not unlike the sun, in that its purpose is to nurture and sustain *all*.

Paul touched upon this point, saying:

"Christ is all, and in all. . . . So we, being many, are *one* body in Christ."

In short, the Christ is the conscious correlation of being between God and man, in whom His kingdom dwells forever.

CHAPTER VII

PERHAPS YOU will ask: what difference does it make that we have the spiritual creation *within* us, and nothing is material? Don't we still have our same problems? And doesn't the world continue in its usual state of turmoil?

Aren't there more diseased and mentally sick people today than ever before, with hospitals and sanatoria literally bulging their walls to care for the ailing? And isn't it a fact that evil and crime and immorality are more rampant than at any time in recorded history?

What are we to think of our once respected institution of marriage, the sanctity of the family tie, crumbling under a spiraling divorce rate? And what about corruption in government, ruthless business practices, the duplicity in human relations, all spreading like the green baytree?

And—but why enumerate more?

Indeed, all this *is* a devastating indictment; yet it falls far short of existing within the jurisdiction of God's domain, notwithstanding all the evidence to the contrary.

It was essentially to prove the falsity of this evidence that Jesus came forward to teach man the truth of being.

There is but a single answer to these seemingly justifiable charges, and it amounts to this: so long as you are disposed to believe that you and the creation are constituted of material substance, then so long will the evils of a material world increase and multiply in your experience.

It is the nature of matter to sow the seed of evil, inasmuch as it is itself a falsity. An effect can be no more substantial than its cause. If you believe in the reality of evil, you cannot escape its destructive effects in your experience. God knows of neither evil nor a material creation; these are wholly your *own* conceptions, and both are erroneous.

It was of evil and a material world that Solomon said:

> **"I have seen all the works that are done under the sun; and, behold, all is vanity and vexation of spirit."**

Man can never look forward to the *millennium,* so long as he looks for it in matter. Materialism, in whichever way you choose to look at it, is unsubstantial, unsatisfactory, and often despairing. In desperation, you will be compelled to turn to God,

> **"Whose peace passeth all understanding."**

Deliverance from such confusion is that simple.

The question will be asked, and reasonably so: why should one's mere belief that man and the creation are material be the source of so much unhappiness, unrest, misfortune and tragedy in the world?

Here you have the core of the whole enigma: *belief.* Belief in error. Belief in that which does not exist, but only appears to be—as Immanuel Kant pointed out—a sensuous *image* of reality.

You externalize your thoughts into material objects in your own consciousness, and then *believe* they are real entities existing outside of yourself. Many of these unreal objects are feared by you, and frequently they become your master. Such fear, and indeed *all* fear, is illusion.

Consequently, it is this belief in things that do not truly exist, but which you fancy are real, that causes you to observe and experience so much distress in the world. If you would but see the truth, that all reality is spiritual and good, your externalized beliefs which you have come to fear and look upon with misgivings would disappear from your consciousness as easily as darkness vanishes before light. This is casting out erroneous belief as Jesus had done.

Job clearly stated:

"Man that is born of a woman is of few days, and full of trouble."

The belief that man is a material entity dooms him, as Job had said, from the very moment that he is born into matter. It is obvious that this is so, since he is merely the image of misdirected thought.

Jeremiah speaks of him, thus:

"Cursed be the man that maketh flesh his arm."

It is plain, according to the venerable Hebrew prophet, that matter is neither the constitution nor intermediary of the real man made in God's image and likeness. His belief that he is material induces the very afflictions that appear to curse him.

Paul puts it in this manner:

"For if ye live after the flesh, ye shall die: but if ye through the Spirit do mortify the deeds of the body, ye shall live. . . . For I know that in my flesh dwelleth no good

thing. . . . For he that soweth to his flesh shall of the flesh
reap corruption."

That matter is an illusion of belief, without any more
substance than the moving image that we observe on the
theatre screen, Paul substantiates, as he adds:

"But ye are *not* in the flesh, but in the Spirit. . . . And he
that soweth to the Spirit shall of the Spirit reap life everlasting."

If you would see your real self as God's conscious image,
you must accept with absolute conviction this paramount
truth: *all*, including yourself, is Spirit and Its spiritual expression.

Once this recognition is firmly established in mind, the
beginning of wisdom has indeed come to you.

Sir Arthur Stanley Eddington declared:

"Mind is the first and most direct thing in our experience;
all else is remote inference."

Is this not what Jesus and his apostles have taught
through precept and parable?

To illustrate, Paul said:

"With the mind I myself serve the law of God; but with
the flesh the law of sin."

If God had created material flesh, could Paul conscientiously have made such a statement?

Hardly.

The kingdom of God can appear to you in no other way
than through mind, for the door by which it enters must,

of necessity, be consciousness, the substance out of which it is made.

Paul particularly stressed this fact:

"Be not conformed to this world; but be ye transformed by the *renewing* of your mind."

By merely a change of thought, the whole kingdom of God can make itself evident to you, while simultaneously the so-called material world will disappear from your consciousness, the only place where it could possibly reside. You do not have to die first to leave this material world and enter into the spiritual one. On the contrary, you need but to see the *truth* in consciousness that you are eternal, and that a material world is nothing more than a sheer *belief* of matter.

It is solely by the *renewing of your mind,* as Paul had stated, that the fallacies of belief dissolve before the light of truth.

Consider for a moment the endless things that man evolves erroneously in his mind when he believes in the reality of material illusion! He is born in the atmosphere of a religious or philosophic belief patterned in matter, yet worships a spiritual Godhead that knows nothing of, and much less could be correlated with, materialism. Thus believing matter to be something, and indispensable to his existence, he covets, hates, resorts to cunning, corrupts, steals, injures and even provokes himself to commit murder, to obtain that which has no substance outside of his own consciousness.

In short, man's whole life is strictly regimented to matter from the cradle to the grave, and still he clings stub-

bornly to the belief that this is the life God had prescribed
for him in His image and likeness.

What else can this depiction be but a caricature of
God's man?

God is infinite love; and, more, He is all that the infinitude of love could possibly imply. This boundless love of
His is wholly spiritual, and could *never* conceive of, let
alone induce, fallacy, disorder and evil.

To absolutely refuse to be identified with any of these
destructive beliefs is the first step in overcoming their effects. This can be done only by identifying yourself with
God, being coexistent with Him. Uniting yourself thus
with God, you enter into spiritual consciousness, and such
consciousness is an impregnable defense against all error.
Being constantly aware that God fills all space, exercises
all authority, and maintains man in eternal harmony, is
your warrant to resist everything unlike good.

Of this sovereignty, Benjamin Franklin said:

**"I have lived a long time, and the longer I live, the more
convincing proofs I see of this truth: that God governs in
the affairs of men."**

Notwithstanding whatever your sense of the material
tells you, you are the spiritual expression of God alone.
Beyond any shadow of doubt, you are as glorious, perfect, eternal and joyous as God; for you are the true image
of these qualities which are His. It is self-evident that if
you are His image and likeness, you could no more reflect
opposite qualities than a mirror could reproduce an ill-
humored expression when your face is creased in smiles. It
is your false beliefs that objectify themselves as the evils
in your experience.

In his sermon on the mount, Jesus exhorted:

"Be ye therefore perfect, even as your Father which is in heaven is perfect."

Surely the great teacher of truth would not have incited the multitude on the mountainside to be something that was contrary to their inherent nature.

Know with intense conviction that you are spiritual and *not* material, that you are indestructible, dynamic, and express glowing health, strength, intelligence and dominion, because these qualities are God's faculties. For in the degree that you spiritualize your thinking, so will you bring these qualities into your being. You cannot be the image or reflection of anything else, seeing that there is *nothing* besides God to reflect.

It was God's purpose that you express Him in unbounded freedom and joy. The design of creation was to *give* you the kingdom.

Think of it! All that is God's is yours. A heritage unheard of. *All* of it yours. What a glorious possession! And to avail yourself of this heritage you need only be aware of it. Feel its spiritual power. Realize the substance out of which it is made. Understand its unfoldment.

Truly you have something for which to shout *halleluiah*. Take it to yourself. Assimilate it. Put it to practical use.

Do not be afraid of God. Embrace Him. Hold fast to the Almighty, and never let Him go. He is *love*. The most compassionate kind of love. Merciful, tender and forbearing.

John, confirming this, said:

"He that loveth not knoweth not God; for God is love."

You coexist with God in His love. He made you to be His witness. His reflection. Yes, He made you to *express* Him in all His glory, to enjoy His sound health, wisdom, abundance, eternal nature. He made you to laugh and be gay, to dance and sing, to be serenely happy.

Said the Psalmist:

"Let all those that put their trust in Thee rejoice: let them ever shout for joy . . . let them also that love Thy name be joyful in Thee."

A long face affected in piety can never be in consonance with the joy His presence inspires. Such piety is likened to the hypocrites whom Jesus alluded to, in his sermon on the mount, as disfiguring their faces.

The fact that the kingdom of God is within you implies that you are spiritually perfect in mind and body, harmonious in all your endeavors, at peace, confident, satisfied, and that nothing whatever can separate you from this grand fact.

When Jesus made this promising declaration:

"Be ye therefore perfect, even as your Father which is in heaven is perfect,"

he knew for a certainty that this transformation was possible of attainment. He knew that this state of perfection was within the reach of all mankind, as Paul later had revealed,

"by the renewing of your mind."

Would the Master have made so amazing a statement if it were not so?

Jesus proved the truth of what he taught by healing the

sick and the sinning. And, more, he assured those that believed in his doctrine that they, too, could do these same works, and added,

"and greater works than these shall he do."

Here hope, quickened by authority, gives fresh impetus to the dreary heart. Healing the sick is the most direct evidence, palpable to the physical senses, that God delivers man from his diseased beliefs.

And why should this be any more incredible today than it was two thousand years ago?

Were we actually physical, we would be without hope; and because we nevertheless *believe* ourselves to be material beings, only makes this much sought-for hope *seem* just beyond our reach.

Paul made it very plain:

"Ye are *not* in the flesh, but in the Spirit."

Virtually all Christendom has wilfully blinded its eyes made deaf its ears, and dulled the understanding of its heart, rather than accept the sublime truth, as revealed by the apostle, that we definitely are *not* in the flesh. Man is purely a conscious idea alone, and abides in Spirit, in the Mind that is God.

If disease is real, and a quality of God's creation, we could never alter this fact even though we were disposed to do so, for we could hardly hope to undo that which He has made. But if disease is unreal, then it is as much illusion as is your material body, and this premise is susceptible to demonstration.

Jesus' healings were based on the proposition that there

is *nothing* else but Spirit, divine Consciousness, and Its innumerable ideas and their activities. This is the *all* of creation, and it exists as eternal thought in the mind of God. Not so much as a speck of anything could possibly have existence outside of this Mind.

Inasmuch as everything in this Mind is perfect and eternal, and you are the image, or reflection, of it—seeing that the kingdom is within you—obviously *you* must be equally as perfect and eternal as that which you reflect. This perfection and eternality is, of course, in the degree that you cast out all materiality from your thought and replace it with the spiritual ideas which you and everything actually are. It is simply a reversal of thought from the material to the spiritual, and clearly seeing this latter picture with mental conviction.

The Master sums it up, thus:

"It is the Spirit that quickeneth; the flesh profiteth nothing."

Your belief that disease is real is to admit that God made it, since it is generally agreed that He made *all* reality; and, too, it admits by the same logic the further belief that you have a real physical body on which the morbid condition acts.

So long as you are predisposed to believe that disease is part of God's creation, rather than an illusion of your material sense of things, the involvement of a diseased phenomenon invariably will be equal to the tenacity and conviction of your belief.

Since God neither created, nor knows of, anything material within His kingdom, mortal man must be left alone to struggle through his illusory existence that both he and the disease are material. Man and a universe of matter are merely misconceptions of the human mind.

If, on the other hand, he would but visualize the nature of his spiritual individuality, the picture of disease would quickly fade into extinction in his experience, because it would no longer have anything of a material character on which to pin its unwholesome appearance.

Whereas your physical body is consciously objectified in your mind, so the disease must have its abode in this self-same mind also. It can evolve its mental purulence and suffering in no other place, since there is no other place for disease to reveal itself.

Well did Philo Judaeus, more than nineteen hundred years ago, declare:

"Ignorance is the cause of disease and destruction."

Were man to look to his Creator for a healing of his malady, he would see the perfection of *all* His ideas, including himself, that make up the kingdom which abides in God's mind; and this exalted conception, steadfastly held in thought—to the exclusion of everything material— annuls the illusion of disease proportionally to the clarity of his discernment.

Immanuel Kant defined this clarity of discernment, which you must look for, in these words:

"If you would see things and ourselves as they are, we should see ourselves in a world of spiritual natures with which our entire real relation neither began nor ended."

This is looking upon God's eternality, and man in His image of it. To see the ideas of God in this true perspective is consciously beholding spiritual creation, the only creation existent. And in the ratio that you persist in retaining this vision of reality in your thought will the illusion of disease disappear from your experience.

The only way to employ spiritual healing is, as Paul had stated:

"to be absent from the body, and to be present with the Lord."

The readiness with which spiritual healing responds is dependent solely upon one's constancy and singleness of mind in this Presence. God *always* is present and conscious of our innermost thoughts.

Isaiah, alluding to the discords of matter, said:

"Thou wilt keep him in perfect peace, whose *mind* is stayed on Thee."

Disease cannot externalize itself on the body without you first outlining its essential nature in your thought.

Job attested to this truism, that the dread of disease ultimately begets disease, when he said:

"For the thing which I greatly feared is come upon me, and that which I was afraid of is come unto me."

Parents unwittingly plant the fear of disease, as they do the seeds of prejudice and intolerance, in the minds of their own offspring, through governing and influencing them by their stronger thought. The immature infant mind is wholly subjugated by the mental atmosphere of its parents, and particularly is this true in the embryonic stage. Your thoughts, no less than your blood and strength, are his nourishment.

To overcome the effects of disease you must reverse the procedure which makes disease evident, and this is done only by mastery of the fear, or evil, that occasioned the disorder. Any inharmony will take flight and disappear the instant you have removed its exciting cause from your consciousness, be it some hidden fear, a persistent resentment for someone, envy, or some such evil thought. This is the type of negative thinking, or ignorance, which Philo Judaeus declared causes disease and destruction.

That we are what we think, and make for ourselves the conditions under which we live, Solomon had long foretold:

"For as he thinketh in his heart, so is he."

Nothing thought, nothing can be wrought. Mere flesh and blood have neither intelligence nor influence to produce phenomena. Thinking alone has this exclusive prerogative.

That this is so, Paul attests:

"They that are in the flesh cannot please God."

This should be an indelible reminder to choose only wholesome thoughts to enrich your mind, as you would similarly select the purest foods to gratify your hunger. For you yourself mold the health and strength of your body, or dissipate it, with the thoughts which you introduce into your consciousness.

Allowing evil thoughts to take possession of your mind induces disease and inharmony, and Jesus expressly verifies this fact, as in the instance when he healed the impotent man at the pool who for thirty and eight years lay bound with his infirmity:

"Behold, thou art made whole: sin no more, lest a worse thing come unto thee."

A word to the wise is sufficient. Disease takes its root in the ignorance of sin and its kindred evils. Jesus made this plain throughout his entire ministry. He never attributed disease to germs or microbes. Germs and microbes are but an elaboration of the lie that man is material.

Fear of disease, the more acute form of ignorance, may readily be removed from your experience by simply laying the axe of truth squarely at the root of this evil.

Nothing *real* can hurt or make man sick, if

"God saw every thing that He had made, and, behold, it was very good."

Moreover, what God had made was equally harmless, while that which He did *not* make evidently must exist only as illusion. So are germs and microbes that supposedly destroy the man that God had made, but merely consume an unreal likeness of him. Clearly discerning this truth, Jesus swept aside all bacterial and symptomatic diagnosis, and healed man through the simple expedient that he is the spiritual and perfect image of God.

If we honestly believe in our hearts the teachings of the Master, that every one of us is capable of doing the works that he has done, and even more, how inconsistent then must we be to look for healing within the ignorance concocted in a bottle called medicine?

From this irrefutable premise it is obvious that God did not make disease, and so it must be unreal. And it is solely this unreality that man fears, an *illusion* of disease which is entirely nonexistent. He fears a morbid picture in his mind that actually is without substance or power, and the most that can be said for it is that it is nothing.

To be more specific, he fears the image of his own

thought, an unreal appearance which he speculatively placed there himself, outlining it as disease and externalizing the disturbance on his assumed material body, which is no less a deceptive appearance than the disease he had outlined in his mind.

The Psalmist was well aware of this destructive belief, but in the realm of illusion only, when he said:

"Yea, though I walk through the valley of the shadow of death, I will fear no evil: for Thou art with me; Thy rod and Thy staff they comfort me."

The Psalmist knew infallibly that life was eternal, established and maintained by God in His mind, and that death was but the termination of the grand illusion that man and the universe are cast in matter. Hence, he had no occasion to fear evil, aware as he was that there was none.

You would never fear evil of any kind either if you but understood the nature of both God and yourself. There is absolutely *nothing* for God's man to fear, and in reality that is the *only* man you are.

You picture images of disease in your mind and call them creations of God, when in fact they are erroneous human beliefs. And this alone is what you fear, your own mental pictures which you have objectified on your mortal body, believing as you do that it is real also. As a consequence, these *miscreations* eventually become your masters, enslaving you to the very beliefs which you yourself have conceived and expanded.

It is the belief that you are a physical entity, susceptible to germs and microbes, that has bound you to disease, and defaced and incapacitated your body. To *know* without the least doubt that your complete existence is purely mental, frees you at once from any so-called external phenomenon, since there is *nothing* physical about you on which to affix extraneous fallacy in the first place.

Fear is an emotion entirely of your *own* making. It has neither place nor sustenance in the divine design. It is wholly mortal. That this is so, Paul substantiates:

"God hath not given us the spirit of fear; but of power, and of love, and of a sound mind."

Fear is akin to poison, and the antithesis of love. To overcome fear, it is essential that you reflect God's power and love and soundness of mind. And when you have fairly made evident these qualities that are His, fear will then have disappeared proportionally from your daily life.

John informs us:

"If we love one another, God dwelleth in us, and His love is perfected in us."

Herein lies the core and nature of the Supreme Being. Not even the love of a mother for her child begins to approach the ineffable love which God has for you.

John then adds:

"There is no fear in love; but perfect love casteth out fear: because fear hath torment."

It is obvious that you cannot cast out reality, therefore fear must be illusory if love can cast it out. It is plain, according to John, that fear is a deceptive intruder.

The noted Dr. J. A. Hadfield said:

"If fear were abolished from modern life, the work of the psychotherapist would be nearly gone."

Dr. Hadfield's assertion indirectly admits fear to be an error of material illusion, else the psychotherapist would be powerless to lend himself toward its elimination. It would be absurd to attempt eliminating that which is real. Fear is removed by knowing the truth about its falsity, and this line of treatment is the procedure resorted to by the successful psychotherapist.

Man has a sensationless body, and this body is compounded of the only substance there is, spiritual consciousness. There is absolutely *no* such thing as matter, not even so much as a grain of it in the entire creation, despite the seeming evidence of it everywhere. Your body and everything you perceive and experience simply *appear* to be formed of matter.

When you feel or see your arm, you merely feel or see your thought which constitutes your arm in consciousness. Your arm thus perceived is no less real because this is so; but, on the contrary, its reality becomes the more apparent and eternal in the ratio that the material arm disappears from your consciousness and the spiritual one appears. In short, the latter arm is always where the former seems to be.

Notwithstanding that both pictures are wholly mental, the spiritual is the real, or God-created, and the material is the illusion.

This fact, that material appearances are deceiving, clearly bears out the conclusions drawn by such outstanding men of science as Jeans, Russell, Eddington and Steinmetz, among innumerable others, that physical things are not what they appear to be.

To quote John Fiske again:

> "Apart from consciousness, there are no such things as color, form, position, or hardness, and there is no such thing as matter."

To illustrate, your real arm can never be injured or defaced by disease or accident. This is so because it abides in the mind of God, and your arms are the image of the only arms of which God has knowledge. So it is with *all* the members of your body, your organs and their activities, of your whole individuality to be exact. Your real conscious body, which is spiritual and the only body you have, is not merely more substantial than your assumed material one appears to be, but it is absolutely perfect and eternal in health, harmony and contentment.

The composition of matter is nothing more than what your mind conceives it to be. Seeing anything as matter is simply seeing a counterfeit, or *miscreation,* of the spiritual idea that God had made. Therefore, when you endeavor to improve the condition of matter with another type of matter, you are attempting to correct something which does not truly exist with something else that has no more reality than the thing it would improve.

To draw an even clearer picture thereof, you are attempting to heal organic matter, which has no knowledge whatever of its own existence, with an organic, vegetable or chemical extract that knows equally nothing of itself, nor what its purpose is to accomplish.

This unintelligible performance of a nauseous draught of medicine administered to the physical body has absolutely no potency of itself to heal. It is solely your thinking, brought into play and manipulated as the strings are in puppetry, that improves or impedes your physical condition. Of prime importance in the development of your illness is your faith, or lack of it, which your thinking mirrors. Indeed, it is the depth of your faith in the medicine that, in the last analysis, heals your complaint of disease or, on the other hand, makes an invalid of you, or worse.

The reputable English medical magazine, *Lancet,* spoke out with high authority on this point:

"Faith and hope . . . are but two of the many mental medicines which a judicious physician may use."

To be sure, faith and hope are the *only* medicines that heal. Material medicine, having no intelligence, can heal nothing. Or to put it another way, the whole business of either recuperation or degeneration takes place in mind alone. Nothing material can possibly exist in God's creation, for

"every thing that He had made . . . was very good."

Every discordant action and appearance of disease on your body has its source and development in erroneous thought, and its entire progression from conception to termination takes place solely in your mind. However, you will perhaps be more inclined to believe that the evolution of the disorder is unfolding on a material body that is separate in substance from this mind, but the fact is your material body is as much an erroneous thought in this self-same mind as is the discordant action or appearance of disease which you have consciously externalized on it.

If this were not actually so, you could never heal disease under *any* circumstance; for it is obvious that if disease is real, God made it, and what He had made no man can efface.

The phenomena of both your material body and the disease only *seem* to be external to your mind; and here let it be indelibly impressed upon your thought that mind is never contained within a brain and skull, but rather are brain and skull mere conceptions of matter in your mind. This is the great departure in your conscious experience where you become the slave, or chained prisoner, of your own beliefs. You blindly believe something that is contrary to reality, and then incarcerate yourself behind its mental bars until freed by the light of truth.

Yet, according to the Master, there are those to whom this liberation never comes. He said:

"Their ears are dull of hearing, and their eyes they have closed; lest at any time they should see with their eyes, and hear with their ears, and should understand with their heart . . . and I should heal them."

It is plain from these words which Jesus uttered that material medicine has no part whatever as a means of healing the body. It is the understanding of the heart, or mind, that disease is an illusion, which wields the power to heal. Material medicine merely encroaches on this power, and takes for itself the credit that rightfully belongs to mind alone.

It is sheer misconception to believe that a material brain is the abode of mind. God alone is *Mind;* and you are the reflection, in consciousness, of *all* that God is, and this reflection is never contained in an outline of matter. The one cannot be cognizant of the other.

That you are the reflection of *all* that God is, Jesus pointed out in his answer to Philip, that he be shown the Father:

"He that hath seen me hath seen the Father."

The image and likeness of God is *all* that He is, and this identity of Him is His witness and expresses Him in *all* His ways.

Every single thing which God has created, its identity, action and continuity, moves within its own designated orbit in His mind. There it resides eternally and perfectly, and its only substance is the consciousness out of which God conceived it. So it is with space and motion, and all dimensional magnitudes. All are mental manifestations in this Mind, and objectified in human understanding through conscious reflection. There are no durational and spatial distances computed from material hypothesis.

To again quote Sir James Hopwood Jeans:

"Ether or space is a creation of thought, not of solid substance."

Whatever appears material always is an erroneous concept of substance in your mind, and such thoughts entomb themselves within everything they create. You reproduce in your mind, although it may appear otherwise, whatever you choose to think, be it disease or health. Every concept which you believe has its origin in brain evolves itself unmistakably in error.

Of the illusion of matter, William Shakespeare said:

"We are such stuff as dreams are made on, and our little life is rounded with a sleep."

To understand reality clearly you must translate everything material back to its spiritual idea, or native origin, as God had created it, and forever holds intact in His mind. Then you will see these objects as they really are.

So did the bard of the Avon see them when he looked more deeply into the truth of being; for then he said:

"There is nothing either good or bad, but *thinking* makes it so."

CHAPTER VIII

LET US endeavor to be even more specific as to this elusive mystery of matter and disease.

Matter is nothing more than an image of thought in your mind. So is a purulent disease manifested as an ulcer on your material body. Both exist only in your mind, and your mind projects its pain, feels its torment, and intensifies or impedes its action. All is within your mind, and subject to its will and authority.

This *all* embraces your body, the ulcer, and the physiological action of the disturbance. And to be more explicit as to the location of the disorder, let us call it a stomach ulcer.

Naturally you will be prompt to reply:

"But I wouldn't want an ulcer; so why should I wish to entertain one in my mind?"

Of course you do not want an ulcer. However, you *do* entertain them in your mind if you believe in their reality, and that they can produce inflammation in all their morbid ugliness upon your body. Not wanting an ulcer, and yet believing that ulcers are real and painful and often enduring, is actually fearing their existence, notwithstanding that such fear may be regarded by you as utterly negligible.

It is this predisposing belief in their reality that conduces to your fear, if not in immediate consciousness, then in its latent state. This fear which invariably is present to a more or less extent, and which you are unable successfully to dispel from your mind despite its seeming unimportance, eventually externalizes itself exactly where the fear resides, in this selfsame mind. There is *no* other place where an ulcer can manifest itself, despite your opinion to the contrary.

And here it is well to repeat the Master's words:

"Ye shall know the truth, and the truth shall make you free."

The truth about the ulcer is that actually it does not exist, despite its seeming appearance and discomfort, because God did not make it; and here, again, let us be reminded that

"every thing that He had made was very good."

From this alone it becomes self-evident that the ulcer is a *miscreation* of your own thinking. Certainly it has no validity or permanence in reality. Obviously it must be an illusion from its first concept to its ultimate evolvement.

You, in turn, become the captive of your own thought projection, and your subsequent fears of what you have conceived oftentimes terminates in anything from chronic invalidism to perhaps death itself. And in the interim, you will have suffered the accompanying displeasure of distasteful diets for perhaps the rest of your natural days, as if God would countenance such incongruity in His perfect creation.

And if you think for a moment that you are *not* a captive of your material sense of things, pray, then, from what else can it possibly be that Jesus promised

"ye shall know the truth, and the truth shall make you free."?

The truth is the fact that you are spiritual and *not* material; and when the light of this verity dawns upon your consciousness, you shall be made free proportionally to the degree of this dawning.

Moreover, these additional words from the Nazarene might similarly enlighten you as to the bondage which your thoughts frequently commit you:

"He hath sent me to heal the brokenhearted, to preach deliverance to the *captives,* and recovering of sight to the blind, to set at liberty them that are bruised."

There can be nothing else to which Jesus inferred you are the *captive* of than your sense of material affliction. Realization of the truth alone exposes the illusion of your erring beliefs.

The senses of a mortal are essentially material; and their physical phenomena explain, because of their impermanence, why a sense of matter must of necessity be mortal. Anything subject to materiality has birth, deteriorates and dies; and this triad of errors exists in the mind that entertains them, and not in a substance called matter.

It should be readily seen that there can be no such thing as matter, if God made His creation from the substance of Himself, Spirit. What you perceive as being matter is but a mistaken sense of its true nature, God's idea, formed of, and subsisting in, the mental substance which constitutes

His mind. Everything that He had made is created out of this same spiritual awareness in which it resides; and this is all that is real and eternal in fact, form, color and composition.

What God had *not* made is evil, and it should be clear to anyone that evil is nothing if, according to John:

"**All things were made by Him; and without Him was not anything made that was made.**"

Assuming evil to be real is equivalent to believing that out of this *nothing* can be made something, the miscreations of illusion.

It should further be clear to the understanding that anything made without Him, and everything in this category must necessarily be evil, exists only as a counterfeit in thought, inasmuch as a mortal can create merely an unreal image presented to his own senses. And this is what you call material and real, or God-created.

In short, this is the illusory product in which you imprison yourself and, in consequence, find yourself to be anything but joyful.

Man in the image and likeness of God is not solely an image of His Person, as is commonly accepted by humankind, but rather is he the image of God's consciousness, in which you and His kingdom abide. This kingdom, in turn, is reflected to your conscious receptivity; for this is the kingdom, His creation, that is within you. Specifically, God's creation is His eternal thoughts transmitted to you, which you see, hear, feel, taste and smell, mentally. There is *no* other way of appreciating reality.

When God made heaven and earth, and all the celestial bodies in the firmament, the cattle and beasts, and fish and fowl, and fruit and herbs of the ground, they became part of Him as His creative and eternal thoughts. Moreover, He alluded to them as an integral part of Himself, as being *one* with Him, according to Genesis:

> "Let *us* make man in *our* image, after *our* likeness: and let them have dominion . . . over all the earth."

Making man in the image of God implies that he is an unlimited partaker of the eternal thoughts which God conceived and maintains for his pleasure.

Plotinus, greatest of the Neo-Platonic philosophers, saw into this truth seventeen hundred years ago; and, out of his inspiring illumination, he bequeathed us these divine facts:

> "External objects present us only with appearances. . . . They are within us. Here the objects we contemplate, and that *which* contemplates, are identical—both being thought. The subject surely cannot know an object different from itself. . . . It is the agreement of the mind *with* itself. . . . The mind is its own witness."

God's ideas are His thoughts, perfect and eternal; and when we look upon one of His ideas, be it a tree, a planet, or a lion, we really are seeing it in our minds while mistakenly believing that it is constituted of matter and exists with its environment outside of us. The truth is that both matter and the phenomena of creation outside of us actually are in our consciousness. Everything is in our consciousness, whether it *appears* outside of us or not. We are the image of God's thoughts, or ideas.

And so, returning to the ulcer, what do you do to combat the situation of a rebellious stomach which your belief alone has occasioned?

You call a doctor.

This, of course, proves that down in the depths of your heart you have greater confidence in the ability of the medical practitioner to heal your ulcer than in God who had created you. And this is not surprising, when we consider that man's fears through the ages have driven him to consort with material means rather than seek his Maker for a healing. The evils of anxiety, alarm and blind tradition, overtaking what was assumed to be an utterly negligible fear, have inculcated in you the further belief that there is no other remedial agency to which you might have recourse, despite what the inspired Psalmist sang:

"Bless the Lord, who forgiveth all thine iniquities; who *healeth* all thy diseases."

After a thorough examination your family physician, reflecting the learning of his alma mater, thoughtfully puts away his thermometer and stethoscope in his little black bag, and efficiently scrawls out a prescription. The formula calls for still another belief in matter, the juice squeezed out of some bitter herb root, fungus extract, or similar preparation, to heal the belief in matter that had originally induced the ulcer.

Since neither the ulcer nor the prescribed remedy have any intelligence to know what they themselves are, or the purpose for which they are to be brought together, yet one is expected to effect a miracle of healing upon the other.

Indeed, such a healing *would* be a miracle far greater than anything Jesus had performed were it possible; but the truth is this: man is a spiritual being and resides in

God's mind, where neither disease nor the material extract of fungus growth or bitter herb root can enter therein. Jesus' healings were accomplished exclusively through mind, never matter. He said, explicitly:

"It is the Spirit that quickeneth; the flesh profiteth nothing."

No one knows better than the honest medical practitioner that you cannot correct the condition of matter by the simple expedient of administering another form of matter. He knows, if his experience has taught him anything, that the patient's faith in the medicine—blind though it may be—is the singular power that heals the sick.

In virtually all his demonstrations, Jesus said:

"Thy faith hath made thee whole; according to your faith be it unto you."

Indeed, the Master did not allude to faith in medicine, for he plainly eschewed *all* material remedies. How much more responsive and effective then shall the answer be to *your* faith when placed directly in God, in whom you "live and move and have your being," and in whom *all* faith imperatively operates?

The sage and beloved Voltaire, influential French writer and fearless reformer, voiced a timely truth when he said:

"Doctors are men who prescribe medicines of which they know little, to cure diseases of which they know less, in human beings of whom they know nothing."

To be sure, doctors and every one else can never know anything about human beings so long as they believe in the efficacy of medicine and the reality of matter.

It is obvious that if the ulcer had its origin in your mind, and it is fairly well established that it can have its existence in no other place, then it must by the same token be expelled therefrom to effect a healing. This is the truth about divine therapeutics, and there can be *no* other therapeutics worthy of the name truth.

Jesus healed disease by casting it out of the consciousness of the sick. He never wrote out prescriptions for medicine, never used a scalpel, nor did he make use of any material method. He knew that the application of such means was impossible to restore health to the ailing. He healed solely through the power of God, and this power is *mind* alone.

The Master made it unmistakably clear that this power was not inherent only in himself, when he said:

"He that believeth on me, the works that I do shall he do also; and greater works than these shall he do."

Such power resides exclusively in God, in His mind, not in medicine, and is reflected to human sense through consciousness. This power, no less than the kingdom of God, is *within* you, seeing that you conversely are *within* Him by virtue of His will.

Let us not deceive ourselves in looking down on the incantations of the aborigines, for we cannot escape the undeniable fact that we ourselves, in subjugating our mentalities to materia medica, are but little removed from the sorceries of the savage, despite our institutions to care for the sick, and the assumption of the medical fraternities that the issues of life and death belong solely unto them, rather than to God.

To those who would arrogate to themselves so great a prerogative, aware as they are of their own inadequacies, it might be well to repeat here these words by Paul:

"If any man think that he knoweth any thing, he knoweth nothing yet as he ought to know."

Of all this so-called material knowledge and idolatry, whether it be in medicine or any of the professions disposed toward matter, the prophet, Jeremiah, declared:

"They are vanity, the work of errors."

Truly, it is your *faith* alone in the preparation labeled medicine that has healed the ulcer, if indeed it has, and not the medicine itself. It is, in effect, one error subduing another, or the greater overcoming the lesser. Your mind, unquestionably, has been the healing agent through your positive belief in the curative powers of the medicine, as it was the causative factor in bringing about the diseased condition on your assumed material body in the first place.

Your doctor and the medical profession, taking full credit for the healing, as though the Creator were dispossessed of His power and prestige, have no such dominion over your mind. Not if you are the image of God, and His kingdom is within you.

It is only when you *surrender* this inherent power to another, as for instance believing in the remedial value of medicine, that you become the captive of error.

This subjection to error was graphically set forth by Paul, who said:

"Know ye not, that to whom ye yield yourselves servants to obey, his servants ye are to whom ye obey?"

The psychology of material therapeutics is mesmeric. It effectuates through human personality and blind confidence a subtle influence over the psychic processes of your thinking. Perhaps no better illustration of this dominance can be found than in the sick patient feeling suddenly well the instant the doctor crosses his threshold, or, conversely, seized with uncontrollable fright. Material medicine *never* effected a real healing.

Benjamin Franklin wisely said:

"God heals, and the doctor takes the fee."

God *always* is the healer, notwithstanding your belief, or the vanity of the medical fraternity.

The kingdom which divine Providence has given to you is not in the province of another to manipulate, much as you are inclined to believe. The power of God is *yours* by reflection, and your faith in this power is the balance that ultimately determines the progress, favorable or otherwise, of the aforesaid ulcer.

No pharmacist can dispense this power to you in a bottle. It is a travesty on the majesty of the Creator to believe that health can be found in a concoction of unpalatable herb extracts, designated medicine, when He, Himself, had created and subsequently sustains you out of His substance to be His image and likeness.

Of this travesty, Dr. Mason Good, Fellow of the Royal Society, and licentiate of the Royal College of Physicians, declared:

"The effects of medicine on the human system are in the highest degree uncertain; except, indeed, that it has already destroyed more lives than war, pestilence, and famine, all combined."

Should your fear of the ulcer meanwhile become greater than what your faith is in the medicine that has been prescribed for you, it is a foregone conclusion that the purulent complaint will become proportionally aggravated in the outlining which you will be projecting on the screen of your mind. And if this be the case, your family physician will be obliged, out of fear himself, to dispatch you posthaste to the hospital. Here a specialist in surgery will be waiting with scalpel in hand to cut open your belief of a material body, so that a more intimate study of the offending disorder may be made.

And should your faith in the prescribed surgery, as in the medicine, likewise fall short of overcoming your mounting fear of the malady, not to mention the added risk of the operation, you will in all probability succumb as a result to death itself.

And this is the hypothesis on which we shall proceed.

From the motivating concept of the ulcer to the final breath which you will have drawn, all has passed in kaleidoscopic review before your mind. There never actually was a material body nor an ulcer. The only thing that died was your *sense* of a material body, and this illusory *sense* is all that will be buried in the ground. This so-called body is the conscious *misconception* which your loved ones erroneously believe contained your spiritual and eternal individuality.

To be more specific, the entire manifestation of your existence from beginning to end was merely a mental picture unfolded in your consciousness, nothing more. *Sensing* it as physical was mistakenly believing that it existed in, and of, matter.

That which is true and God-created, for all else is a false *sense* of His creation, can never die.

Jesus plainly stated:

"If a man keep my saying, he shall never see death."

Yet, on the first of the following month, when your surviving family pays the doctor the bill for his services, he will tell them with humility that he had done all that medical science could do for you, although it was the operation itself that had cut short your mortal existence. And more, he will perhaps take them into his confidence and explain that yours was one of those hopeless cases beyond the help of this science, as if that could be any solace to those you left behind.

As a matter of fact there is *no* such thing as medical science. It is an imposition on the divine laws of reality to believe that there is. The sciences confirm only the *truth* in God's creation, and by the widest stretch of the imagination pure science could never admit of such fallacy and sheer presumption as materia medica.

George Bernard Shaw aptly declared:

"The rank and file of doctors are no more scientific than their tailors. Doctoring is an art, not a science."

Were the profession of medicine a science, there certainly should be no such amount of guesswork in its application, nor hit and miss diagnoses, trial and error treatment, and diametrically opposite results from the same remedy on identical disorders.

It is generally those that have distinguished themselves in medicine, knowing full well the inconsistencies of their chosen profession, that have outspokenly disclaimed the accepted belief that materia medica is scientific.

Such a one is Dr. Leo M. Davidoff, Professor of Clinical Neurological Surgery at Columbia University, who said:

"Unfortunately, clinical medicine is *not* an exact science."

Indeed, it is not. Nor is it a halfway science. And what is not an exact science is no science at all. The fact is materia medica does not, and cannot, so much as even *approach* science. It has appropriated the name of science, but without its power and validity. Believing that to be real which is material illusion obviously cannot be scientific.

The famous Dr. Harvey Cushing, internationally-known brain surgeon and teacher, is even more emphatic:

"As a matter of fact, it will be a great shock to laymen to learn that a great part of what is called scientific medicine is a fetish and wholly *unscientific*. . . . The practice of medicine is an art and can never approach being a science."

And if this celebrated surgeon, whom lesser practitioners regard with preeminence, has not made himself clear, he puts it still another way:

"Every drug a doctor administers and every operation a surgeon performs is experimental in that the result can never be mathematically calculated. This is far from making medicine a scientific calling."

Dr. Cushing, like all men who have sought after the truth, speaks out of the many years of his practical experience.

Had not God made His creation faultless? Or had He blundered in its construction, and then found Himself compelled to call on an illusion of His image, man, to keep in repair that which He was unable to perfect?

This is the travesty of matter, imperfect man endeavoring to improve his imperfection.

Shortly before the hour set for your last rites, the family pastor appeared for a friendly call on your bereaved kinsfolk, and compassionately informed them that

"the Lord giveth life, and the Lord taketh it away,"

when not so many Sundays before he preached in your very presence, and with all the conviction and eloquence which he was able to summon forth, quoting as he did the Master, that

"this is life eternal . . . and whosoever . . . believeth in me shall never die."

This was something over which to really be concerned about, were it possible of course for you to be concerned at this stage of the transition. But assuming it were so, you will by this time have become so confused as to what this whole business of life and death is anyway, that it will be all you can do to keep from turning over in your grave and resigning yourself to the destiny from which no traveler returns.

First, it was told you almost from infancy that life is eternal, and secondly, the kingdom of God is within you, while thirdly, dominion over *every* thing is ever yours; and here they have planted you in the cold ground and lowered a heavy marble slab on top of you. To be sure, it is all so inconsistent, and disconcerting, that you are almost glad to be lying exactly where your loved ones have laid you.

And, besides, you have likewise come to the conclusion that the whole province of materiality from birth to death is absolutely beyond all reason, mercy and understanding anyway, what with everyone along the way from maternity delivery room to the undertaker holding out a hand to collect a fee as you pass by in the parade of mortal existence.

Such is the drama of material illusion.

This is not so of yourself, however, in spiritual reality. If you would heal yourself, and come into eternal life through "knowing the truth that makes you free," you must reverse the whole process of a *sense* of everything being material, and realize through this same medium of mind a *sense* of it being spiritual, or real.

This conversion can only be experienced, as Paul had revealed, if

"ye be transformed by the renewing of your mind."

Since everything that God had made is forged out of His substance, divine consciousness, there can be but *one* means of cognizance and appreciation, and that is through realization. Your senses are of the same mentality as that from which you frame your thoughts.

Everything resides, assumes identity, and has its peculiar functions, in mind, from conception of the embryonic idea to its unfolding activities and final fulfillment. This applies not only to what is real, but to the physical illusion as well, since the latter is a mental misconception of the former. Therefore, to free yourself of the ulcer you would simply *unsee,* in consciousness, the unreal appearance of the disorder, and in its place *realize* the perfect body that you have through spiritual reflection, immune from any semblance of disease.

This is experiencing reality, seeing through the material counterfeit and thus beholding the truth.

Until you consciously *feel* this spiritual regeneration taking hold on you, you can never truly know

"the peace of God, which passeth all understanding."

There is one thing that disease or discord of any kind cannot long withstand, and that is a constant and earnest seeking of your true status as the child of God, resident in His mind. Whatever may be your problem be assured that it will disappear proportionally to the sincerity of your *conscious* presence in Him; for it is

"in Him we live, and move, and have our being."

Disease, or any inharmony, feeds and grows only on the thought which you provide for its subsistence. These evils can have neither origin nor development except through the agency of your thought. When, conversely, the mind is inclined to dwell solely on God, the disease or inharmony no longer has anything to sustain it, and so naturally it begins at once to disintegrate and disappear.

Disease, like sin, vanishes when thought is thoroughly convinced of its spurious nature.

God's consciousness is *your* life. There is no other life. Indeed, God is the *only* consciousness existent, and it is in this consciousness that you have your substance and being.

If the aforesaid ulcer is real, then God made it, and it would be absurd to think that you could remove it, any more than you could remove any other reality and activity which He had made. But if it disappears into its native nothingness, through your mere realization of the truth, then this simple demonstration should be ample proof that it never truly existed in the first place, except as illusion.

This is the absolute basis on which the Master's healing mission was established. Its fundamental principle is that God is *all,* and this *all* irrevocably exists in perfect harmony in the mind of God, not as matter, but as spiritual idea. All else obviously is physical misapprehension.

This is the infallible truth which Jesus successfully interpreted and demonstrated, and left for you as a priceless legacy to "do likewise."

There can be *no* other explanation for his healings. This power to heal the sick, the lame, blind, demented and the sinner, who are with faith, is as much with us today as it was in the days when Jesus trod the dusty roads of Galilee.

To rid yourself of the ulcer, or any other malady of the flesh, you first must determine its cause, which usually is some latent or immediate fear presenting itself as disorder, and this you cast out of your consciousness. This is all Jesus *ever* cast out of the sick, fear of the erroneous thought maintaining the ailment. He never cast out anything of a material nature, because there is nothing of a material nature that can be cast out. It is simply a *sense* of something material that is cast out.

Occasionally, it is necessary to probe deeper than the fear itself in order to cast out the motivating thought responsible for the disorder. Invariably, this proves to be some form of resentment, sin, or just plain ignorance. In these circumstances, Jesus found it imperative to entreat the Father, as when he healed the young man that was lunatic and sore vexed, and whose evil spirit the disciples were unable to cast out. Said he:

"This kind goeth not out but by prayer and fasting."

The Master was hardly alluding to abstinence in this instance, but rather to the spiritual profundity required to effectively see man in his *oneness* with God. He saw the lunatic in his perfect state, as God had made him in His image and likeness, and this inspired vision healed him.

The tremendous faith which the sick had in Jesus, wherever he abode, was in itself casting out their afflictions.

Once you clearly see this truth and likewise cast out of your consciousness the exciting cause of your disorder, that will be the end of your ulcer, or whatever may be your anxiety. Let it ever be known that disease or inharmony of *any* kind never comes to you by way of floating germs or other material phenomena in the atmosphere, but from erroneous thought wafting through the realm of your own consciousness.

The physician, looking on matter as real substance, is concerned only in material effects. He can cut out the ulcer, to be sure, that is to say the illusion of it; but so long as he is unaware of its cause or true location, it will continue to reappear on the sufferer's so-called body in the degree that the sufferer harbors its reality in his mind.

Humanity generally is ignorant of the fact that the exciting cause expressing itself as disease on your body is simply fear in its manifold forms and aspects.

The eminent medical research authority, Dr. Alexis Carrel, to again quote him, confirms this truth:

"When envy, hate, fear are habitual, they are capable of starting genuine diseases. . . . Man, as known to the

specialists, is far from being the concrete man, the real man. . . . In fact, our ignorance is profound."

Dr. Edward Weiss, another respected member of the medical fraternity, makes this conservative estimate on the subject:

> **"After one hundred seventy-five years of medical darkness, we are emerging into the light as to the source of about fifty per cent of humanity's ills—a state of mind."**

If fifty per cent of humanity's ills, as Dr. Weiss declared, emanate from a state of mind, with all its envies, animosities, fears, malice, and the whole gamut of evil, from where then comes the other fifty per cent?

From the *same* state of mind, of course.

There is *no* other place from where illness can come. *All* disease has its inception and development in mind. It is just another figment of the belief in matter that a material body is susceptible to microbes. Cast out this belief instantly from your mind, that *anything* can be material, even an amount equal to the half-size of a microbe's whisker.

Well did Confucious say:

> **"An angry man is *always* full of poison."**

Disease either is in the province of matter or it is in mind, certainly not in both. Mind and substance matter have no affinity one for the other. It is only a question of time until it will be universally accepted by mankind that the body inherently is in mind, as is the microbe, and everything observable to consciousness.

Believing that disease is real in man is to admit that the image of God can be afflicted, which obviously implies the imperfection of the Creator, Himself, seeing that man is made in His express likeness.

By abandoning from your thought the material *sense* of God's image as suffering from an ulcer, and at the same time realizing through your spiritual *sense* that you are the perfect and conscious likeness of God, is casting out the erroneous belief of disorder.

As Paul had pointed out,

> "be ye transformed by the renewing of your mind, and be not conformed to this (material) world,"

if you would have the seeming ulcer pass out of your experience and the likeness of health, which is God's true image, appear.

Indeed, you are not giving up anything real, but rather a mortal or illusory *sense* of it. You are as perfect and healthy as your Creator if you are made in His image and likeness.

The truth of being will unfold simply and clearly to your understanding, and in your experience, provided of course that you hold this perfect conception of yourself persistently in thought. You must hold it to the exclusion of any adverse material suggestion attempting to gain entrance to your mind. You must ever be on guard, and alert, before the holy sanctum of your thought; and keep these instigating evils, or erroneous trespassers, out of your consciousness as you would thieves and murderers from your home.

This is casting out the belief of disease, which is unreal, and realizing in its place the truth of being, which is perfect, eternal, and ever available. When this is done with solid conviction, and an abiding faith in God, the ulcer, or whatever might be the claim of inharmony, will disappear as readily as mist before the sunlight.

To illustrate God's unerring healing power with a concrete example of its application, the author recounts his own experience with a critical disease from which reputable specialists in the medical profession declared there was no hope of recovery.

My distress, on learning of this prognosis, was inexpressible.

Afflicted, as I was, with pulmonary tuberculosis that had progressed to a far advanced state, there apparently was no alternative left to me but accept this authoritative verdict that I was doomed to die.

It was in the darkness of this despair that the light of truth burst upon me. It so happened that I was thumbing casually through the Bible, which was left at my bedside by a friend in the spirit of helpfulness, when I came upon this enlightening citation by Christ Jesus:

"Ye shall know the truth, and the truth shall make you free."

This startling statement was the spark of hope that dawned upon my forlorn thought as I stumbled those last days through a wilderness so dark that all seemed irreparable unto my soul.

I pondered this passage long and searchingly. Its simply stated assurance held out to me so bright a promise that I was thoroughly satisfied I had found the divine *staff* on which to lean through this trial. And, more, I was sublimely inspired by the character and power of the man who had uttered these encouraging words that awakened my dormant understanding to the infinite possibilities implied therein. And being thus awakened, the light of his presence touched me to the pith of my being.

As a result of this experience, a faith that was real, absorbing, and alive, overwhelmed me.

It should be disclosed here that my friend, who had left the Bible with me, laid the groundwork for this transformation by first quoting the citation to me, among others, in hopes that I might be freed from the destiny which my moribund beliefs were objectifying. Incidentally, I listened to her with the forbearance characteristic of those about to depart for newer pastures, assuming that these reassuring Scriptural passages were for the obvious purpose of lifting my spirits for the impending hegira that awaited me.

Although I knew this lady to be an able metaphysician, I regarded her interpretations of these several quotations as utterly transcendental, and impracticable. But the seed, for all that, had not fallen on barren soil; seeing that, some days later, while thumbing through the Bible on the aforesaid occasion, this powerful passage by the Master stood out in sharp relief before my receptive eyes. It radiated a promise of hope so profound, the likes of which I had heretofore never so much as suspected.

This was the cup of cold water that had borne much fruit.

I sat up in bed and immediately began to pray, something I had seldom ever done before, imploring God to give me the understanding to absorb these truths which Jesus was endeavoring to expound in the synagogues, along the wayside, in the desert, on the mountainsides. I wanted—oh, so much to live, to recapture my health again, to run and play, to dance and swim, sing and laugh, to do the things I loved and dreamed about, to know that I was actually alive once more, as God had intended I should be.

And this was what I had learned through that "still small voice" which came to me as the Christ from God: if the *truth* could make me free, then it was self-evident that I was the captive of truth's antipode, error, or my affliction. And it was only by *knowing* the truth that I could hope to be free of this error to which I was captive. Inasmuch as *knowing* is solely mental, the ray of light that had that instant flashed across my consciousness informed me that I was bound in thought, alone, to the disease that was rapidly consuming me.

It was obvious that, from this premise laid down by the Master, the *truth* definitely would free me from the belief of tuberculosis that I was entertaining in my mind, together with its unfavorable progress and inevitable termination. By correcting this belief with the truth, through the simple medium of my thought, as one would a mistake in arithmetic, I could by this mere expedient have my health restored.

Incredible as this seemed, nevertheless here was the truth literally begging—as always—to be accepted.

With this scintilla of a new day unfolding in my mind, I was firmly convinced that I was already being transformed to health; and, to facilitate this healing, I promptly summoned my friend for her help in the further study of the Master's teachings.

And this, I quickly learned: there is *nothing* existent that is material. Everything that God had made was created out of the substance of His own consciousness, including myself, and this substance is wholly mental in composition, structure and dimension.

I saw the entire picture of reality unfold before me, if not in its most distinct phase, then at least observable; and, seeing it thus, I had but to deal henceforth with enlightened thought exclusively.

I was fully satisfied that I had come upon the divine truth, as Jesus had expounded it, and my next step was to apply it to the ends for which it was conceived.

I shall never forget that day, the surge of faith that swept through me, and the conviction that I was started on the road to recovery, and no longer need fear the imminence of death. It was like being unburdened from a colossal weight. Although I had unwittingly bound myself, as if with chains, to an unreal belief called tuberculosis, I was now thoroughly convinced that the healing power of truth pouring into my consciousness would free me from its dire effects.

I was so inspired and divinely carried away by this glorious discovery that I was unable to keep myself longer in bed, although I had not risen from it for months on end.

My recovery was rapid, bewildering the physicians that had attended me. Moreover, it was a complete healing.

Looking back on this experience, two things in particular stand out that have impressed me deeply. They are *persistence* in your course and an *unalterable faith,* notwithstanding the seeming odds against you, that God will answer your prayers for health if you but seek Him in Spirit with the full confidence of your heart.

Isaiah confirms this:

"Thou wilt keep him in perfect peace, whose mind is stayed on Thee: because he trusteth in Thee."

Such must be the quality of your *persistence* and *faith* if you would bring to yourself divine healing; for according to the sincerity of your heart will your prayers be answered. And should your healing continue in abeyance for an unreasonable time, this should intimate that you be even more steadfast in your perseverance and stronger still in your faith, since the situation implies that the deep-seated nature of the disorder in your consciousness requires but greater confidence that God will answer you.

And here James counsels us:

"Let patience have her perfect work."

To illustrate further the power of *persistence* and *faith*, draw an imaginary line across your mental vision, and *under* this line place your problem, whether it be a critical disease, impoverishment, unhappiness, or whatever may be your lot. Then *above* the line establish God.

Now take your stand, mentally of course, and cling to God with all your strength of heart and mind, with *persistence* and *unalterable faith*. Strive to keep your thought ever *above* the line, on God alone, and never allow it if possible to fall *below* it, thereby dwelling on your problem, or error; and, if your fidelity to Him is half the sincerity of your purpose, you cannot help but triumph over your problem.

It cannot be repeated too often, nor too strongly, that by keeping your mind steadfastly on God, you are refusing to feed the disorder, or error, the least whit of mental nourishment on which it must thrive to subsist. Disease or inharmony of *any* kind has both its inception and evolution only in the thought which entertains it.

Were there no thought to promote disease and discord, disease and discord would be nonexistent. And fearing what you yourself have conceived obviously increases its involvement in the ratio to the intensity of the fear. All is in your thought.

Conversely, by keeping your mind stayed fast on God, as Isaiah had exhorted, impoverishes the very nature of the disorder owing to the lack of mental sustenance to maintain it. Meanwhile, as your mind absorbs the influx of His spiritual power and perfect health, the disease or inharmony disappears from your experience proportionally to the light of *truth* unfolding in your consciousness.

It is that simple.

The truth is applicable in *any* adversity or crisis. To but realize that our bodies are the conscious reflection of the One perfect body that exists eternally in the mind of God, and to hold firmly to this truth with *persistence* and *unalterable faith*—while excluding all material error that would gain entrance to your thought—will dissolve any disorder that is unlike God's perfect man.

This is precisely the way God *intended* it should be. By keeping your mind stayed on Him is realizing your true self, your perfect self, exempt from all disease and discord. This is having faith.

Solomon put it this way:

"For as a man thinketh in his heart, so is he."

You absolutely are what you think; and it behooves you to think only the truth, if you would be robust in health and well-being.

Marcus Aurelius summed it up thus:

"Our life is what our thoughts make it."

Diseased thoughts, or error, beget their own peculiar characteristics, a diseased body. Such are the immutable laws of error.

"There sat a certain man at Lystra, impotent in his feet, being a cripple from his mother's womb, who never had walked: the same heard Paul speak: who steadfastly beholding him, and perceiving that he *had* faith to be healed, said with a loud voice, 'Stand upright on thy feet!'"

And the impotent man immediately leaped and walked.

CHAPTER IX

THE PROFESSION of medicine from Hippocrates to the distinguished Benjamin Rush of our early American colonial period, and on up to present-day therapeutics as pursued by Alexis Carrel, has been little more than an ingenious play on the minds and credulity of humankind. The practice of medicine, considered in its most favorable light, is merely another and more pretentious form of mesmerism.

It is related in the Bible that

"Asa . . . was diseased in his feet, until his disease was exceedingly great: yet in his disease he sought not to the Lord, but to the physicians; and Asa died."

Modern medicine, with all its speculative discoveries and burnished instruments with which to probe the human body, has advanced over primitive forms of treatment only in the organization and propaganda of its closely-knitted fraternity. Disease has multiplied enormously since Asa chose to place his faith in the physicians. And increasing with this multiplicity has been the creation of new-born ailments which have plagued mankind from the day that Hippocrates wrote out his first prescription nearly twenty-five hundred years ago.

These new diseases, conceived, stamped with identity,

and propagated through fear by the medical faculty, subtly perpetuate this most dreaded of all errors in the fertile soil of the human mind.

The fear of disease together with its erroneous antidote, the belief that the material body can be healed of its morbidity with matter, enhances the appalling influence of disease.

So long as materia medica persists in introducing diseased thoughts and their kindred fears into the human mind, inventing frightening names for new bodily disorders and delineating their terrifying symptoms, disease will surely continue to multiply in still differing forms. This is the nature of error.

It is apparent that the general run of medical practitioners know little, or care nothing, about the consequences which the disclosure of disease and its symptoms engender, fanning itself to destructive heights in the minds of both themselves and the layman. And think not that the practitioner is immune from such fear. It is only when the disease is in his patient that he is unafraid of its dread.

Man's immemorial fear of disease, his constant mulling over it, comparing it with other forms of disorder, enlarging upon it through his impressionable thought, speculating upon its ultimate development and destructive possibilities, is infallibly the progenitor of disease.

This is so particularly in the case of the layman who fancies that his physician is endowed with an esoteric knowledge for healing the human body that is little short of the wisdom belonging to divine Providence. Had he rather less faith, or confidence, in the practice of medicine and its practitioners to heal the body with matter, the less likely would he become the victim of disease.

The practice of medicine is not only far from being the answer to man's great anxiety, the healing of his discordant body, but it definitely is the foremost propagator of disease.

In striking contrast to the pretensions of the medical profession, Jesus made it clear throughout his entire ministry that God alone is the healer. And this power, said he, is within yourself, seeing that His kingdom is within you.

When we place our trust and hopes in the medical practitioner and his remedies, are we not rather paying lip-service to the Master, who had taught and demonstrated the healing truth for all posterity to emulate?

Jesus never carried a medicine bag on his rounds among the sick. He never administered drugs nor resorted to any surgical operations in effecting his healings. Yet he healed the most inveterate maladies, the kind the medical fraternity would label hopeless. And he healed them spontaneously, proving incontrovertibly that medicine has no power to heal. Nor did the Master's patients require prolonged periods for convalescence, such as is the custom today, notwithstanding that a large number of them had been impotent and deformed from birth.

But more remarkable is the fact that this great teacher of the *truth* made it plain that you and I are capable of doing these very same works which he did; and then he added:

"and greater works than these shall you do."

Were this not possible of achievement, certainly Jesus would never have addressed his disciples, thus:

"Heal the sick, cleanse the lepers, raise the dead, cast out devils: freely ye have received, freely give."

Indeed, it was not medicine bags filled with ill-smelling drugs that the disciples received from the Master when he told them to heal the sick; but it was rather the *truth* which they dispensed to the ailing, the truth that frees man from the shackles of his diseased beliefs.

Jesus instructed his disciples to

"heal *all* manner of sickness and *all* manner of disease."

It is clear that he did not school these simple fishermen and tillers of the soil in materia medica to do this healing, but in metaphysics. They did not write prescriptions to be compounded by apothecaries, although apothecaries flourished then as they do today. The teachings of Hippocrates at that time had been thriving for four hundred years.

What a counterfeit must materia medica then be when exposed to the light of reality, as demonstrated by Jesus in both his healing and teaching!

Either the Master's method of healing is the true one, and the practice of medicine false, or it is the other way round. Certainly both methods cannot be sound.

Weighed upon the scales of reason, materia medica becomes an imposture to the unsuspecting human mind.

It is, as Jesus had bluntly stated,

"a lie, and the father of it."

Although Hippocrates, the father of medicine, was born some four hundred years before the Master, his well-entrenched works, and those of his pupils, were annulled "in the twinkling of an eye" by the mere introduction of the truth which Jesus taught and successfully demonstrated.

What, then, it will be asked, has become of this healing truth?

Obviously, it had been left in the hands of those few disciples guiding the destiny of the early Church in Corinth, Galatia, Ephesus, Philippi, to name but several among the more important centers of religious life before the Church as we now know it was established. But after a few centuries this early Church apparently had compromised with the resurgence of materia medica, particularly during its renaissance under the Greek physician-philosopher, Claudius Galen, a worthy successor of the astute Hippocrates. Seeing that it had gradually lost the essential faith to heal, and no longer could effectively demonstrate the power of truth, the Church as much as said to this medical fledgling that was swiftly encroaching within its ecclesiastical province:

"Here, we'll turn over to you the business of healing the body of disease, and we'll confine ourselves exclusively hereafter to saving its soul. There's more than enough for both of us to keep busy by such an arrangement."

With this decadence in the early Christian Church, much of the true spiritual quintessence which Jesus taught and left for humankind to practice was lost.

Scarcely anything is known of either Hippocrates or his assumed writings. Considerable medical lore has been attributed to him, but all of it is without the slightest authenticity. The greater part of these manuscripts were ascertained to have been first written as much as six hundred years or more after his death.

The so-called Hippocratic oath is likewise conjectural, wherein the profession of medicine is specifically identified as an *art* rather than a science. Incidentally, much can be said for this oath in its original entirety, whoever its author might be, the irony being that comparatively few members of the medical fraternity adhere to its principles anyway.

Just what conclusion Hippocrates himself might have drawn as to the ultimate value of materia medica, posterity shall never know.

However, Dr. Benjamin Rush, surgeon-general of the Continental army, signer of the Declaration of Independence, and notable American pioneer in, and teacher of, medicine at the University of Pennsylvania, left a most emphatic opinion on Hippocrates' contribution to mankind. Said he:

> "His account of the heart, the brain, the senses, the intestines, and organs of generation, is so replete with absurdities that it would be disgusting to mention them. . . . His physiological opinions are fanciful. . . . It is impossible to calculate the mischief which Hippocrates has done by first marking Nature with his name, and afterwards letting her loose upon sick people. Millions have perished by her hands in all ages and countries."

Such is the conclusion arrived at by this highly respected teacher in medicine after a lifetime of matured reflection, based on the experience and observation of an extensive practice.

Of present-day therapeutics, Dr. Alexis Carrel, eminent in the field of pathological research, reveals this interesting challenge to the unfounded claims of materia medica:

> "Medicine is *far* from having decreased human sufferings as much as it endeavors to make us believe. . . . In spite of the progress achieved in heating, ventilation and

lighting of houses, of dietary hygiene, bathrooms, and sports, of periodic medical examinations, and increasing numbers of medical specialists, not even *one* day has been added to the span of human life."

This appraisal by Dr. Carrel is particularly enlightening when it is considered that he has been associated with the foremost men and women in both the United States and Europe in the work of medical research.

The fact that "not even one day has been added to the span of human life," as Dr. Carrel's intensive studies at the Rockefeller Institute for Medical Research have revealed, contradicts the many loosely circulated statements that man has added fifteen to twenty years to his existence on earth, thanks to the advances made in medicine.

Here, again, the Master's ringing rebuke fittingly applies to all such misleading propaganda, whose source is in the medical fraternities:

"When he speaketh a lie, he speaketh of his own: for he is a liar, and the father of it."

The truth is this: the statistics apparently are correct, being based on the actuarial figures of the life insurance companies; but, indeed, this does not signify that the average man who had succumbed in the year 1900, at the age of 65, would have lived to be 80 years were he to pass away today. The increased age in question applies almost exclusively to infant and early youth periods, its gains being greatly responsible for the over-all picture in which these statistics are solely concerned.

The proof of this conclusion is borne out by the United States Department of Health, National Office of Vital Statistics, and every insurance company in America.

The explanation for this survival of the infant and early youth periods are many, and not the least is the fact that public antagonism toward overdosing and exhaustive medication at these tender ages have considerably conduced to a lowered mortality figure. Babies were literally decimated until only recent years by this overzealous dosing.

To bear out Dr. Carrel's researches, a Metropolitan Life Insurance Company statistician disclosed this interesting information in regard to increased longevity:

> "Many periodicals have, I believe, publicized the fact that the average length of human life, sometimes referred to as the expectation of life, has increased substantially during the last fifty years. . . . The term *span of human life* has usually been used in the sense of the ultimate length of human life. There is no evidence in mortality statistics that the ultimate length of human life has increased appreciably in modern times. This agrees with Dr. Carrel's statement."

To delve deeper into early statistics, in contrast with those of today, brings to light the unmistakable fact that it is equally the economic and living standards of infants and childhood that has reduced the mortality rate among this age-group, while obviously increasing the life expectancy of the whole. To twist these figures and say the older portion of the population is increasing its life span fifteen to twenty years is either a wilful distortion of the facts or plain ignorance.

The Actuarial Division of the Prudential Insurance Company of America adds to this confirmation:

> "As Dr. Carrel has pointed out, there is no evidence that the life span has changed to any material degree within historic times."

There are an incredible number of people who actually believe that the medical fraternity through alliance with the pharmaceutical manufacturer have concocted preparations in bottles, or otherwise, that will add no less than a dozen years to your life. Our newspapers and periodicals, and not a few erudite dupes, are daily being exploited through the subtle means employed by commercialism to disseminate these fallacies.

The New York Life Insurance Company contributes this pertinent information to clarify the subject:

"The expectation of life at ages beyond 60 is little different from that of one hundred years ago."

These statistical calculations are arrived at by the several insurance companies themselves, and it is their business that they be actuarially correct. The publicized statements that the average length of life has increased simply means that a greater proportion of people in this country survive infancy and childhood, and thereby tend to live out a larger *part* of the life span.

Cleanliness and child welfare, particularly sanitation improvements in congested areas, have contributed considerably toward this progression.

It is obvious that the quaffing of noxious drugs played no part in this natural evolvement. It was plainly social progress rather than medical fable that conduced to this increasing proportion of people living out a larger part of their life span. Man lives no longer on the average in his later years today than he did fifty, a hundred, or a thousand years ago. It is the immature period in life that accounts for this increase, and not the older portion of the population.

Were there any basis that materia medica is the salutary influence promoting the health and longevity of man, surely the medical fraternity itself should be the shining example of this claim. But, according to a recent edition of the *Statistical Bulletin,* official publication of the Metropolitan Life Insurance Company, we learn:

> **"The mortality of American physicians as a group is essentially the same as that for the white population in general."**

If statistics can therefore be a criterion, the unlearned layman might well assume the role of medical adviser to his physician without the latter faring any the worse for it.

That this is no play upon words, nor statistics, the well-known Dr. William S. Sadler, Professor of Physiologic Therapeutics at Chicago's Postgraduate Medical School, stated:

> **"It is generally believed by experienced physicians that at least two-thirds of the ordinary cases of sickness which doctors are called upon to treat would, if left entirely alone, recover without the aid of the doctor or his medicine."**

Can any practicing physician honestly say that this is not the fact in his daily experience among the sick?

And who would be so bold as to say that a goodly proportion of the remaining third would not equally recover if left entirely alone?

Sir John Marshall, Fellow of the Royal Society and Royal College of Surgeons, Professor of Surgery at University College, addressing the London University Medical School, said:

> "*The Vis medicatrix naturae* (the healing power of nature) is the agent to employ in the healing of an ulcer, or the union of a broken bone; and it is equally true that the physician or surgeon *never* cured a disease."

Dr. Marshall, laying bare his experience and observation of a lifetime, unites with the conviction of the metaphysician that God alone heals, and that materia medica does nothing toward the cure but collect the fee. When will humankind awake to this fact?

The fetish of medicine has through the years subtly infiltrated the province of man's better judgment, while increasingly exercising dominance over his mind by engendering the virus of fear.

The famed Dr. Thomas Sydenham, regarded by his contemporaries of a bygone era as preeminent in the field of medicine, said:

> "I often think more could be left to Nature than we are in the habit of leaving to her. To imagine that she always wants the help of art is an error, and an unlearned error too."

If man would have more faith in Nature, and less in medical art, he could depend *entirely* upon her.

Molière, whose studied observations into the errors of medicine have been widely recognized, declared:

> "Nearly all men die of their remedies, and not of their illnesses."

If certain foods can cause attacks of indigestion and poisoning, what sort of miracle do you expect to take place by pouring into your distressed system the vile and

noisome concoctions from which your physician would re-
coil under similar circumstances?

Your problem, by so dosing yourself, becomes greater
still, and not infrequently disastrous; for in the last analysis Nature alone must do the healing despite the ill-
advised aid of your well-intentioned doctor.

Dr. Marshall Hall, respected English practitioner, substantiates this common practice of dosing in the instance of
treating helpless babies:

> **"Of the whole number of fatal cases of disease in infancy,
> a great proportion occur from the inappropriate or undue
> application of exhausting remedies."**

Little wonder then that infancy has had less than half
a chance for survival when, at the first sign of disorder, it
was dosed with the most loathsome concoctions unto
death. Mankind would be rocked to its very foundations
could it know the number of lives that have been stifled
through drugging alone.

Molière's indictment of the medical profession, along
with other bold reformers carrying high his torch through
the years, had sounded a tocsin that is still being heard and
respected in the medical schools to this day. These unsung
stalwarts have contributed more than might be suspected
to the fact that an increasing proportion of people, specifically newly born babies, are today living out a larger
portion of their life span.

Before the turn of the century, Dr. Oliver Wendell
Holmes, Harvard professor of anatomy and physiology,
practicing physician in Boston, and honored with degrees
from Oxford, Cambridge and Edinburgh, among other

famous schools, spoke out before a distinguished medical society:

"I firmly believe that if the whole materia medica, as now used, could be sunk to the bottom of the sea, it would be all the better for mankind and all the worse for the fishes. . . . Every noxious agent, including medicines proper, which hurts a well man, hurts a sick one."

Dr. Holmes, it might be well to mention, had been held in the highest esteem by the American medical profession when he uttered this outspoken stricture.

The practice of medicine has not changed appreciably in those few decades since Dr. Holmes wrote out his final prescription, nor in five times their number. The fact is it has scarcely changed from the primitive methods employed by Hippocrates and Galen, except of course for the addition of a few burnished instruments which now give the ceremony of diagnosis a greater aura of mystery.

To this very day the same nostrums and acrid draughts, though differing in nomenclature, taste and composition, are still being dispensed to a credulous public. For without the blind belief that exists in these unpalatable formulas, the profession of medicine would be more dead than the countless corpses that have succumbed to their depleting action. No one knows better than the medical practitioner that the more loathsome the taste of the apothecary's concoction, the greater is the patient's faith in the ingredients.

The same is true as to the price of the prescription; for the higher its cost, the more the patient evaluates the worth of his doctor's judgment. It is upon this train of gullibility that materia medica flourishes like the green bay-tree.

According to the Associated Press, one Albert Marthaler, color expert for the Arner Company, a large drug producing firm in Buffalo, N. Y., has directed the coloring of 29-billion pills and tablets of some 2,160 shades and tints. Although the public, says Mr. Marthaler, prefers white pills over all other colors, second choice is in the various shades of red. The public, he adds, is sensitive to the slightest change from the color they are used to in the pills they buy.

Think of it! 29-billions of pills and tablets manufactured and sold by a *single* firm!

Both Life Magazine and Reader's Digest revealed in recent issues that Americans alone take 3,360,000,000 sleeping pills a year, an approximate average of 24 for every man, woman and child in the country.

While a leader in this same drug field disclosed the fact that more than 11,000,000-pounds of aspirin is taken every year just for headaches.

Indeed, this is a mimicry of the Creator's wisdom to believe that a jot of health can be regained through use of the whole lot of them.

The multi-billions of pills produced by *all* the drug firms in this country alone is enough to stagger the imagination. And still this mighty Niagara of tinctured pellets is but a fraction of the medicinal preparations offered for sale, what with virtual rivers of its fluid counterpart, together with powders and unguents, all of which a deluded public drugs itself.

The famed Sir William Osler, internationally-known

medical educator, speaks from personal experience on the subject. Said he:

> "The desire to take medicine is perhaps the greatest fea-
> ture which distinguishes man from animals. . . . He has
> an inborn craving for medicine. Heroic dosing for sev-
> eral generations has given his tissues a thirst for drugs. . . .
> Even in minor ailments, which would yield to dieting or
> to simple home remedies, the doctor's visit is not thought
> to be complete without the prescription. Now that the
> pharmacists have cloaked even the most nauseous reme-
> dies, the temptation is to use medicine at every oppor-
> tunity."

On another occasion this respected physician and medical teacher of two continents declared:

> "For generations the people of the United States have
> indulged in an orgie of drugging. Between polypharmacy
> in the profession, and quack medicines, the American
> body has become saturated *ad nauseam*."

When Sir William Osler sought a scapegoat on which to
pin the sins of materia medica, he boldly stated:

> "The medical profession has no more insidious foe than
> the larger pharmaceutical houses, threatening to become
> a huge parasite, eating the vitals of the body medical.
> We all know only too well the bastard literature which
> floods the mail, every page of which illustrates the truth
> of the axiom, the greater the ignorance the greater the
> dogmatism. Much of its advertisements of nostrums are
> foisted on the profession by men who trade on the inno-
> cent credulity of the regular physician, quite as much as
> any quack preys on the gullible public."

Here is a clear admission by a renowned medical educator that proves incontrovertibly that the doctor knows no more what he is doing when writing a prescription than does the patient of what he is pouring into his system. It is tantamount to Jesus' declaration:

"The blind leading the blind."

What with the latest antibiotic drugs, almost everyone frequently reads about and personally knows of cases within his knowledge, where the patients using them have died, barely escaped death, or became invalids from their effects. Indeed, this is a widespread condition, attested by every medical journal. All antibiotics are produced by living organisms, especially a bacterium or fungus growth, a fermented mold or mildew—in other words, plain putrefaction or rot. And this is what you accept into your blood stream.

In the instance of Dr. Oliver Wendell Holmes, he was merely revealing to the medical profession what he sincerely believed to be the practice of educated ignorance. He made bare an honest and courageous conviction that came from the depths of his heart. He simply wished to bring to light, notwithstanding its far-reaching consequences, what the accumulation of his many years of medical knowledge and observation had taught him. His higher sense of reason, and divine truth, told him that something more logical than inanimate matter must surely be man's only recourse to health.

Consequently, it became rather obvious to him that the truth which heals, and likewise blesses all mankind, could never be found in a medicated pellet, nor in a bottle of nauseous liquid.

The great number of honest physicians and surgeons that could today conscientiously reecho this distinguished Harvard professor's conviction, were it convenient to bare their true sentiments without jeopardizing their livelihood and standing in their respective communities, would astound humankind.

Dr. Norman Barnesby, practicing physician and author of Medical Chaos and Crime, discloses one of countless shocking incidents, which by no means is uncommon among members in the profession:

"A well-known physician, an acquaintance of mine, whose reputation in New York is of the best, told me recently that his great success in medicine was not due to any unusual skill or knowledge, but to the fact that he 'knew when to take advantage of the other fellow's ignorance.' "

Notwithstanding that the profession of medicine generally is made up from as fine a class of men and women as are to be found in any vocation, this does not imply that materia medica is the divine expedient for restoring health. Were all the graveyards and catacombs from the past to testify in behalf of the medical victims prematurely laid to rest within them, exposing the wilful malpractice, stupidity and ignorance of those licensed to practice medicine free of restraint, civilization would at long last be shaken loose from its age-old apathy.

So long as the qualifications for entrance to a medical school are solely the wherewithal to finance a course of instruction, regardless of the moral and humanitarian fitness of the student, so long will the profession of medicine be infested with such examples of evil as Dr. Barnesby had pointed out. It is no longer a secret today that the choice of a medical career is influenced far more by its pecuniary rewards than any desire to be of benevolent service to humanity.

Nor is it an exaggeration to say that many a practicing physician today has been literally pushed into his present vocation more to please the wishes of a doting mother than himself.

Dr. George W. Wagoner of Johnstown, Penn., delivering the President's address before the Pennsylvania Medical Society in Philadelphia, and published in the New England Medical Journal, said:

"If the mighty host of those who have been rushed into untimely graves by incompetent, pretending physicians could be marshalled into an army and marched in ghastly review before the astonished eyes of our indifferent legislatures, what a ghost-like multitude of outraged victims there would be, one which would appall by its magnitude and horror, and excite the lawmakers to a frenzy of action."

Has there been any honest and concerted action by the organized medical fraternities, in its pronounced greed for the dollar, to counteract this obvious slaughter?

None whatever. This would be an admission of its fallacy. It is far more expedient to bury its errors with the bones of its victims.

Little wonder that the reputable Dr. Mason Good was constrained to graphically proclaim:

"The effects of medicine on the human system . . . has already destroyed more lives than war, pestilence, and famine, all combined."

Explaining to a victim's bereaved loved ones with a sad shake of the head, notwithstanding the deceased's healthy glow and stamina, that his case was hopeless and beyond help, absolves more malpractitioners daily than is ever suspected.

The guilty should, by all means, be taken into custody and placed behind bars like any other malefactor. But where powerful pressure groups, such as the medical profession, influence and shape the laws of our government in their behalf, who passes judgment on such offenses but the malpractitioner himself? The old moss-covered stock phrase, "beyond the hope of medical science," condones every act in the lexicon of manslaughter.

Dr. Harold L. Foss, Fellow of the American College of Surgeons, and surgeon-in-chief of Geisinger Hospital, Danville, Penn., wrote in the *Bulletin,* official publication of the American College of Surgeons:

> **"An urge to operate, whether indications exist or not . . . is being too frequently experienced by many of our recent graduates. . . . Lack of surgical judgment and technical skill are accounting for an enormous amount of unnecessary hospitalization, invalidism and, all too frequently, fatal terminations. The gravity of this state of affairs is well known to most older surgeons. Unless this condition is corrected, some day the public will find it out, when it will in all probability offer its own solution. . . . Any doctor who possesses a state license, which by no means of the imagination is any evidence of surgical ability, can without a semblance of restriction take into his own hands all the other lives he may wish, and continue to do so as long as he can find a gullible public willing to follow his advice. The condition is widespread."**

What means has the public to protect itself, seeing that dead men tell no tales?

Merely by knowing the truth that materia medica is human error.

It was precisely such a state of affairs within the secretive cloisters of the medical fraternity that prompted the sage English writer, George Bernard Shaw, to declare:

"Every doctor will allow a colleague to decimate a whole countryside sooner than violate the bond of professional etiquet by giving him away. . . . Anyone who has known doctors well enough to hear medical shop talked without reserve knows that they are full of stories about each other's blunders and errors."

The excessive power which the medical organizations have arrogated to themselves gives both authorization and impunity for legal murder to those licensed within their membership. This tremendous power is not only tied in with our schools of higher learning, but reaches deep into the apathetic legislative chambers of state and federal governments.

Whereas any layman would be hailed before a criminal court and his life demanded by an outraged medical profession for the identical crime perpetrated by a duly licensed practitioner, the latter need only swear that he had killed in the interest of science to win immunity from both the court and the medical societies. The solicitous non-professional, in no less an honest endeavor to succor his fellow man lying in distress, must in all likelihood pay the supreme penalty because his similar efforts were in vain, while not so much as a shadow of guilt is cast upon the licensed malpractitioner for the same offense.

The power behind such legal immunity is the well-known political influence of the combined medical organizations, instituted with all the cunning and subtlety of which material thinking is capable. As an example, a supine humanity has long been indoctrinated by this school of thought with the belief that this influence actually is put forward in the public interest. This is but one of the soporifics out of the medicine bag of materia medica to pervert your thinking.

Dr. Roy H. McKay, Fellow of the American College of Surgeons, rose up in vehement protest over this shameful abuse of privilege. Said he:

> **"The fact that any man with an *M.D.* after his name is permitted to explore to the far frontiers of medicine and surgery, leaving behind the victims of his ignorance, is something that concerns the thinking profession more than it cares to admit."**

The euphemistic phrase, "ethics of medicine," which we often hear mentioned, is a tacit obligation to suppress the repeated blunders and errors, as well as the immoral and criminal practices, within the membership.

Dr. Dean Lewis, Surgeon-in-chief of Johns Hopkins Hospital, and also Professor of Surgery at Johns Hopkins University in Baltimore, minced no words when he declared:

> **"The bane of modern medicine is a merciless commercialism."**

And why should this be surprising?

If the practice of medicine is honest, its commercial aspects should be no different than that of any other pursuit. But the truth is this, and Dr. Lewis has unmistakably alluded to it: the practice of medicine is being exploited for the express purpose of enriching the licensed practitioner. And herein lies its great evil, considering that today we have an incredibly increased amount of indiscriminate medication and cutting up of the human body, to the detriment of the patient's health and pocketbook.

It is this merciless commercialism, which Dr. Lewis points out, that is the motivating force behind the excessive power of the medical interests. This organized power, in league with the huge pharmaceutical houses, is constantly being used to drive out of existence any competitive agency that would allay pain and suffering. This autocratic pressure is skilfully exercised through press, radio and television campaigns on the pretext of protecting the public health, but this is hardly the fact. The medical profession's antagonism to other forms of healing is displayed for the sole purpose of monopolizing the commercial aspects alone of this ever expanding and lucrative field.

The master minds that guide the destiny of materia medica have gone so far in their crusade to stamp out opposition, that they have even attempted to suppress the divine teachings of faith healing as taught by Jesus, the greatest of all healers. Their attacks on other methods of healing have been merciless, and steeped in calumny where it was necessary to serve the ends of their purpose. The medical fraternity has virtually demanded, not unlike any other illegal monopoly, that the province of healing the sick body be restricted wholly unto its licensed members.

Dr. James H. Means, President of the American College of Physicians, has strongly censured such dictatorship:

"At the present time the electorate of the American Medical Association is apathetic and inarticulate. . . . It is allowing the medical politicians to run things about as they please, and official spokesmen . . . hurl their thunderbolts of wrath at all who differ with orthodox doctrine."

This merciless commercialism in medicine, particularly in the branch of surgery where the larger fees tempt the unscrupulous practitioner to greater and more dangerous use of the scalpel, is a far cry from the divine power of God, who had made us perfect, and will keep us so if we will but turn from the idols of matter and recognize our spiritual heritage.

Ironically, the Church, in whose domain the healing of the sick appropriately belongs, unwittingly gives aid and comfort to the medical fraternity in its encroachment upon the province that is manifestly her own.

Are we not told in Exodus:

"I am the Lord that healeth thee."?

If it is true that God does the healing, of what avail then is the doctor? And his medicine?

The Psalmist, too, exhorts us:

"Bless the Lord . . . who healeth all thy diseases."

It is little wonder that disease has multiplied in the ratio that we have looked for the power to heal in matter, rather than in God.

Occasionally one of the electorate will rear up and break the traces of professional ethics, as did Dr. Graham Lusk, Fellow of the Royal Society of Edinburgh, in an article exposing his fellow practitioners, and published in the Journal of the American Medical Association:

"We are all dollar chasers and intellectually deficient; and the truth of the whole matter is that the (medical) system is rotten and reeking, and cries out for drastic reformation. . . ."

In an authenticated article published in Woman's Home Companion, under the title of *Unnecessary Operations,* by Albert Deutsch, this generally-known traffic in surgery was bared:

"Medical men have long known the shocking fact that many of the nine million surgical operations performed annually in America are unnecessary. Among doctors it is an open secret that in many an operating-room the cloak of surgery covers mayhem and even manslaughter. The time has come for the public to know the truth. Hardly an organ of the human body is safe from the menace of needless surgery. An impressive array of leading doctors attest the fact. Every year thousands of anatomical parts from tonsils to stomachs are cut away or taken out for any one or a combination of reasons—faulty diagnosis, overzealous surgeons, incompetent or mercenary doctors, fee-splitting conspiracies or an inexcusable surrender to the morbid wish of some patients to be cut open."

This shameful condition becomes even more appalling when it is openly admitted by virtually every practicing physician and surgeon.

A noted practitioner told Mr. Deutsch:

"Excessive surgery will be curbed successfully only when the victimized public demands it strongly enough."

Can a more disgraceful indictment be visualized than this outspoken admission by a prominent surgeon of the medical fraternity?

Herein lies the over-all error, stripped to its core. The public mistakenly believes the panacea that leads to health is outside of themselves, in matter, or medicine, when the truth is this: *all* is in themselves, in their own consciousness, where both the illusion of a material body and the disease reside.

Mr. Deutsch continues:

"Today there are too many surgical mistakes, too many surgical crimes. There are too many unqualified doctors cutting up the human body with impunity, literally getting away with murder in the operating room. There are too many operations motivated more by an interest in the patient's pocketbook than in his health. . . . Vain and neurotic patients, sloppy diagnosticians and mercenary surgeons have combined to make appendectomy the biggest surgical racket of all time. . . . The sound physician knows that no surgical operation, minor or major, is without some element of danger."

It might be well to add here that whatever invites any element of danger to life or limb cannot be of divine origin. It is the product of human invention, and wholly untrustworthy.

Consider for a moment the implications which nine million operations in a year suggest! How many of this incredible number are prematurely shunted off each year under tombstones can only be conjectured.

Numerically, every man, woman and child in the United States undergoes at least one operation approximately every fifteen years. In a lifetime this conservatively averages no less than four for every inhabitant, provided that the use of operative treatment is not further increased. However, if the figures from past years can be considered a fair base for future calculation, the number of operations that will mount in the years to come shall be in the precise ratio that medical ignorance, fear, and the belief that the scalpel is a healing agent, predominates human thinking.

What a lucrative industry these astronomical figures prove the branch of surgery alone to be! These statistics, when reckoned from a monetary point of view, and particularly where avarice consorts with fear, are the Midas touch of the medical profession, which surely must disquiet the long sleep of the Phrygian king.

We are quick to throw up our hands in horror over the barbarous practice of vivisection on dumb animals, yet close our eyes to the fact that millions of human beings— guinea pigs all—are blindly being sacrificed daily to the scalpel merely for pecuniary consideration.

This indictment of surgery as practiced today is upheld, in the same article in Woman's Home Companion, by the reputable Dr. Leo M. Davidoff, attending Neurological Surgeon of New York's Montefiore hospital, who said:

> **"Mr. Deutsch is absolutely correct in his statements. . . . While it is my sincere hope that unnecessary surgical operations will in the course of time be reduced to a minimum, I am pessimistic over the possibility of ever wholly eradicating them."**

This venality and wilful disregard of human life runs through the whole gamut of modern medicine, proportionally more today than ever in the history of civilization, notwithstanding the many honest and conscientious practitioners within its fold. Such sordid practice, indulged in by the disciples of materia medica, has been chronicled since ancient times; and so it will always be in the future, and greatly multiplied, so long as man puts his faith in man and matter rather than in God alone.

If, as Jesus has said:

"The Son can do nothing of himself, but what he seeth the Father do,"

what physician or surgeon actually believes that his hit and miss, or trial and error, treatment is that what he "seeth the Father do"?

Neither physician nor surgeon can change *any* condition of the human body; the patient's thought alone makes and changes its own condition.

All through the Master's career as a teacher, he taught and demonstrated that only God can heal us of our diseases, in so far as we have faith "as a grain of mustard seed" in His ability to do so. He distinctly said that the flesh *profiteth nothing*.

Why was Jesus disposed to speak so lightly of the flesh when humanity, on the other hand, literally worships it?

The answer is a simple one: flesh, as matter, is nothing more than an erroneous belief in the human mind. It is merely an image of thought in your consciousness. There actually is no such thing as fleshly matter, or matter of *any* kind. If this were not so, Jesus could never have healed the blind, the lame, the leper and the impotent, solely through realization of the truth that man is not material but spiritual.

This explains the error in which the practitioners of medicine and surgery inextricably involve themselves. Believing that matter is real, they invite greater and more dangerous experimentation in this illusory belief. Eventually, the initiate finds himself implicated in, and condon-

ing, malpractice; and, as a consequence, he allows himself
to be drawn into its mercenary aspects of commercialism.
The worst offenders become conscienceless, and encourage
the delusion that the dangers of the scalpel are negligible.

That such dangers are negligible are contradicted by
any responsible practitioner.

Dr. Max Thorek, widely-known Surgeon-in-chief of the
American Hospital in Chicago, Professor of Surgery in this
country's foremost schools, and a Fellow in many American and foreign medical societies, said:

> "In the art of surgery error is more likely to occur than
> in almost any other line of human endeavor. . . . No
> surgeon, no matter how skilful or proficient he may be,
> should ever consider himself beyond the possibility of
> error or accident. . . . The first great error in surgery is
> unnecessary operation, and the next is the undertaking
> of a major operation which the surgeon is not technically
> fitted to perform. It is well known that both these errors
> are *common* in this era of unlimited surgical operative
> interference."

So long as matter is believed to be real substance, the
train of evil consequences resulting from this belief will
be in direct proportion to the intensity of your conviction
in material existence. Error, whether it emerges from the
surgeon's scalpel or the bricklayer's handiwork, always is
rooted in the illusion of matter, never in spiritual substance. The seed of materialism can only beget its own
kind, error.

Where monetary consideration is the incentive of the
practitioner, Dr. George F. Butler of Chicago, in an article
published in the American Journal of Clinical Medicine,
said:

"The *commercialism* of treating a patient unnecessarily, of taking advantage of his misfortune to frighten him into being treated indefinitely or operated on unnecessarily for the sole purpose of extracting a little more money from him, is not business; it is downright *dishonesty*. The physician who prostitutes his profession by frightening and then literally robbing the sick is a more contemptible robber than the footpad."

The question arises: if matter is not real, how then can there be any danger to it through the errors and commercialism in which materia medica interests itself?

The answer is a simple one: so long as man believes he and the medical treatment are material, he obviously will suffer the dangers and errors of this illusory belief in the degree of his conviction in it.

Where the illusion of matter is believed to be real substance, there can be no line of demarcation as to how far a doctor may safely probe into the condition of his patient; for conscience is an unpredictable factor in assuming risk where the other fellow's life is concerned. The most unconscionable practitioner frequently believes himself to be humanitarian and benevolent right up to the final breath of his patient.

To believe that medicine and the scalpel are man's salvation in the healing of his body, after considering the spectacle of unrestrained but legal drugging and butchery taking place daily in our homes and operating rooms across the country, is to question the wisdom God brought forth in conceiving His image and likeness.

There is but one absolute way to regain, or retain, your health, and that is to clearly see and realize the *truth* that man is the conscious image of his Creator and exists eternally in His mind along with everything else that He has created. This priceless knowledge, seen and felt with profound conviction, is the sole basis and power which heals. This is the secret of Jesus' demonstrations.

To illustrate again the curative power of truth, the author recounts another experience of a chronic condition of bleeding hemorrhoids terminating in insufferable constriction.

Taken reluctantly from a hotel in a strange city to the hospital, surgeons prescribed an immediate operation. Notwithstanding the excruciating pain which I was undergoing, I insisted on conferring first with my metaphysician friend whom I introduced in the preceding chapter. The surgeon in charge gravely advised me that time was a serious matter in my case, and that further delay was inviting the almost certain development of malignancy, if such a condition already was not apparent.

It was not enough that I was in constant agony, but this well-meaning surgeon planted the seed of a second fear in my mind besides. It became imperative that I uproot the thought of malignancy at once. Here I was, suddenly, with twice the problem than when I was brought to the hospital, the constricted hemorrhoids and the added fear of the appalling consequences which an indiscreet doctor tactlessly outlined in my consciousness. And to make this anxiety more burdensome, my metaphysician friend was not immediately available, owing to the fact that I was several hundred miles from her home.

I took my stand none the less, and stood my ground resolutely on the side of God.

When finally, a couple days later, my friend came to see me at the hospital, she emphatically declared that the surgeon was *powerless* to cut out anything that God had made.

I also was reminded by her of what Solomon had said:

"Whatsoever God doeth, it shall be for ever: nothing can be put to it, nor any thing taken from it."

It was evident that if I was God's image and likeness, nothing diseased or otherwise could be put to it, nor cut away from it.

Jesus, too, alluded to this fact:

"Which of you by taking thought can add one cubit unto his stature?"

Or conversely, who, by taking thought, can *take away* one cubit?

Clearly and immediately, I saw the truth that man *is* perfect, and that the protruding and bleeding hemorrhoids, despite their painful constriction, was wholly an illusion of matter. The only thing that the surgeon could possibly cut away was a *belief* of a condition that appeared to exist physically. Everything God had made, including every *part* of His image and likeness, is eternal and beyond man's power to destroy, injure or cut away.

The last vestige of fear disappeared that instant from my consciousness and in its place I experienced, as Paul had said I would,

"The peace of God which passeth all understanding."

The pain quickly vanished, and my recovery from the distressing condition was similarly rapid. I left the hospital, without benefit of either operation or medical treatment, completely healed, notwithstanding that I had been plagued with this affliction for many years.

The hospital staff was utterly taken aback by this perfectly natural healing, an acute pathological condition responding to the healthful currents of *truth*.

Everything in this kaleidoscopic study, the hemorrhoids, surgeons, scalpel, the fear of malignancy, all was an erroneous thought structure in my consciousness, and I had but to cast out of it the entire distasteful picture and see the truth of my perfection to regain complete harmony.

It might be interesting to reveal that this divine demonstration gave impulse to still another, the overcoming of chronic constipation. It took simply the same enlightening truth, clearly seen and realized, to understand that God never created constipation any more than He had made the other afflicting conditions that are the lot of mortal man. All that He had made was *good,* and from this premise it was evident to me that constipation must merely be an erroneous *belief* of physical inactivity.

God's law is *eternal* activity, and peristalsis cannot be impeded in His image and likeness. The belief of inactivity mirrors the belief of a body constituted of matter, and both are illusions without any semblance of reality.

By steadfastly refusing to recognize the claim of inactivity, knowing as we should that God's image and likeness is *always* perfect, activity has got to express itself, as it definitely did for me. This eternal *truth,* ever manifesting itself, is *the miracle that heals*.

As a result, there has been no recurrence of the constipation, nor of the chronic hemorrhoids; and discarded permanently were the nauseous cathartics and purgatives that once seemed so essential to my existence.

This is a concrete example of what a changed belief will do, despite the nature, intensity or gravity of one's affliction. This change of belief is simply to look away from error, which is merely spurious thought, and realize the gentle but engulfing power of truth that is ever available to your receptive consciousness. God is love, and every bodily organ and activity which He has created is constituted in, and of, this love.

Always remember that your belief that God's love has ceased being active, in all or part of your body, is the damaging concept responsible for starting the belief of inactivity.

"For as he thinketh in his heart, so is he."

A positive response imperatively must come to *every* disordered organ or function of the body, notwithstanding the type and involvement of the malady, when the mind is earnestly fixed on God and the truth of His creation. Great numbers of people everywhere are witnesses to this fact, particularly those foredoomed hopeless by materia medica.

Did not Jesus say:

"He that believeth on me, the works that I do shall he do also; and greater works than these shall he do."?

It is without saying that the Master employed neither medicines nor scalpel to effect his healings, but *truth* alone, the truth that man is spiritual and lives solely in mind, and not in matter.

By availing yourself of ever-present truth, spiritual consciousness, you also can effect these same healings consummated by the master of all healers.

The ceaseless fads on how and what to eat, the value of saturating the body with vitamins, enzymes, medicinal tonics, and their like, which only enriches the pocketbooks of those prescribing and preparing them for sale, would be humorous indeed were it not that a gullible public actually believes in their efficacy. There is no more health in manufactured foods prepared with these substances than in medicines. Even the numerous medical publications have at long last been obliged to expose these obnoxious commercial practices and exhort the public to cling to natural foods, eschewing the fads of modern manufacture. God *never* made a food that lacked the substance to promote health.

It has become a farce, if not an affront to the intelligence of mankind, when almost any doctor will, for a price, indorse any manufactured food, cigarette, toothpaste, soap or mattress, as conducive to the health and well-being of the consumer. But the absurdity of it all is that he does this with a deep sense of authority, when the truth is he knows no more about the products which he has indorsed than the public whom he unwittingly hoodwinks.

Cornelia Otis Skinner, brilliant actress and writer, gave utterance to a timely truth when she said:

"The only time I ever have indigestion is when I eat so-called health foods."

Were it not for the fear which the medical profession inculcates in the public mind, together with the credulity in most of us, virtually all the doctor's *éclat* would vanish overnight. For such individuals as have been educated in the belief that a draft of fresh air will bring on a deathly cold, scarcely any physician would be so indiscreet as to prescribe ventilation and jeopardize a lucrative practice.

Right you are, immortal Voltaire, in assailing error with this self-evident truth:

"The art of medicine consists in amusing the patient while Nature cures the disease."

The increasing number of ingenious reminders through press, television, radio, and similar mediums, to the effect that you see your doctor at the first ache or pain, has been bringing more fear-laden business into medical offices than a first-rate epidemic. And not a few of these aches, which would readily pass away of themselves through the processes of Nature, have been buried with the bones of such trusting folk as have been beguiled by these dismaying catch-phrases.

In its annual survey of seven thousand member hospitals in the United States, the American Hospital Association reports that over 20,000,000 patients were hospitalized last year. This is one out of every eight persons in the United States confined to a hospital bed, and does not include those in non-member hospitals, nor the undeterminable millions foregoing hospitalization for various reasons, and choosing to suffer it out in peace at home. Without reckoning these latter categories, it amounts to approximately twelve per cent of our population. Such figures come near identifying ourselves as a nation of hypochondriacs, and yet we are told that we have not nearly enough hospital facilities to take care of our increasing number of sick people.

It is little wonder that there is a growing demand within medical circles to curb unnecessary treatment and hospitalization. Gaining the attention of the mind's receptive faculties incessantly with thoughts of disease, and their involvements, obviously multiplies the volume of it as surely as persistent advertising increases merchandising sales.

There would be far less headstones in our graveyards because of premature death if American surgeons emulated the famed Dr. Albert Theodor Billroth, Viennese surgeon, who said:

> **"Before deciding on the necessity of an operation, I always propose to myself this question: would you permit such an operation as you intend performing on your patient to be done on yourself? Years and experience bring in their train a certain degree of hesitancy."**

If operations conduce to make man well without further endangering his life, why set up a borderline as to how far one may safely probe with the scalpel? Operations either are a good thing in prolonging life or they are, conversely, a pernicious practice. Only a headstrong materialist would attempt to find a happy medium.

Few surgeons of sound mind, including the eminent Dr. Billroth, once a bold and reckless operator himself by his own confession, would permit ninety per cent of the operations being performed on others to be done on themselves under similar circumstances. Surgeons will tell you the reason for this is that they are inherently cowards, but such a pretext is nothing more than a bald-faced evasion of facts. The admission of cowardice is merely a cloak to conceal the truth which hard experience has taught them, that surgery is a downright dangerous business.

Man, putting his trust in a surgeon's hands rather than

in God, when his life is at stake, might well consider first the advice of Isaiah:

"**Cease ye from man, whose breath is in his nostrils: for wherein is he to be accounted of?**"

It is a simple matter for any surgeon, when a patient succumbs solely from the effects of his knife, to write down in his report, *unforeseen complications*. This brief notation covers a multitude of sins, yet it is rarely made out in expiation of a surgeon.

Where the lust for money is a foremost consideration in weighing a decision to operate, few surgeons in this materialistic age can be expected to heed Dr. Billroth's example of hesitancy in the use of the scalpel.

Disease, as well as other forms of disorder, can be eliminated only through the processes of the mind. The same holds true as to the *cause* of inharmony. So long as the human mind is constantly bombarded with the fear of disease, as it admittedly is through the press, television, radio, and by word of mouth, disease will continue to increase, until a mental defense is set up to intercept it. The propaganda of disease is both its seed and fertility.

Hardly a better example of this revealing truth can be had than in the current increase of cancer and heart disease keeping abreast of their expanding propaganda through the last few decades. The endless reminders of these afflictions directed to the public mind, the only medium qualified to harbor them, tend to beget their likeness through the very fear that is broadcast.

When will humankind finally recognize, and stamp out, this open cesspool of contagion?

Dr. Harvey Cushing substantiates this transmission of disease outlining itself in the human mind. Said he:

"There is a tradition among surgeons that they are likely to meet their end by the same malady in the treatment in which they have themselves specialized."

Here is an instance of fear *already* in the making.

If this is true of the surgeon, who has imbibed all his knowledge of medicine through the agency of mind, why expect tranquillity of mind from the layman who fears *all* that the surgeon knows.

Did not Job confirm this fact, when he said:

"The thing which I greatly feared is come upon me, and that which I was afraid of is come unto me."?

Were the mind truly understood instead of being taken merely as an adjunct of the body, disease and all inharmony would disappear from your experience as easily as moisture vaporizes in sunlight. Each little ache or pain, which prompts you to run post-haste to the doctor, has its entire genesis and unfoldment in your mind, even to the externalization of it on your body, which likewise is in this selfsame mind.

The doctor himself can do absolutely nothing toward removing it. You *alone* must do this if it is to be removed. And you, of course, unwittingly do it through your *faith* in him to destroy it. All is accomplished through mind, despite what you or the doctor might think to the contrary. Were you disposed to place a mere jot of this same faith in yourself to do the job in the first place —seeing that the kingdom of God is within you—the doctor soon would be pursuing another vocation.

Sir William Osler, speaking with authority solely for the ears of his medical colleagues, lifted the mask free from the face of materia medica and revealed the whole picture of its gigantic deception. Said he:

"Without faith, man can do nothing; with it, even with a fragment, as a grain of mustard seed, all things are possible to him. Faith in us, faith in our drugs and methods, is the great stock and trade of the medical profession. It is the *aurum potabile* (potable gold), the touchstone of success in medicine."

This confession by the distinguished Canadian physician and teacher is the more striking when weighed in the light of his acknowledged skepticism in medicine alone to heal.

If faith is the great secret to healing, the prerequisite to the *aurum potabile,* why then is it not as effectual when practiced in conjunction with sorcery as in materia medica, or better still *in* God?

Dr. Osler continues:

"The psychical method has always played an *important,* though largely unrecognized, part in therapeutics. It is from faith, which buoys up the spirits, that sets the blood flowing more freely, and the nerves playing their part without disturbance, that a large part of the cure arises. Despondency or lack of faith will often sink the stoutest constitution almost to death's door. Faith will enable a spoonful of water or a bread pill to do almost miracles of healing when the best medicines have been given up in despair. The *basis* of the entire profession of medicine is faith in the doctor, his drugs, and his methods."

This is a clear rejection of the Scriptures, that we put our faith in man and drugs rather than in God alone.

Heed these exhortations:

"Bless the Lord . . . who healeth all thy diseases! Cursed be the man that trusteth in man!"

If one is to derive any comfort whatever from Dr. Osler's observations on materia medica, aside from its admitted dependence on faith, it is this: the mind plays not only an important part in the healing of disease, but the *entire* part. The profession of medicine is an obvious imposture, taking for itself the credit, prestige and glory which rightfully belong to mind, much as the sorcerer is venerated for his miraculous gifts of healing although the transformation actually takes place in the pagan consciousness.

If, as Dr. Osler says, the basis of materia medica is faith in the doctor, his drugs, and his methods, then the colossal imposition which medicine has foisted upon the unsuspecting mind is even more clearly seen in its contradistinction to the Master's dicta:

"Have faith in God! Ye cannot serve God and mammon!"

Withdraw the element of faith, which the medical fraternity would appropriate from God and transfer to inanimate matter, and the art of medicine would be left with no more power to heal than the amulet worn by the superstitious tribesman.

What affinity could faith possibly have for inanimate matter?

The prominent medical educator, Dr. George W. Crile, Fellow of the American College of Surgeons, and Professor of Surgery, School of Medicine, Western Reserve University, speaks with more than a little authority on this important subject:

"We can understand the power of . . . faith in one's own
physician, which undoubtedly plays a part in the successful outcome of most therapeutic measures . . . since whatever dispels worry and uncertainty helps to stop the body-
wide activation which leads to lesions as truly physical
as a fracture."

If this be the case, would it not be far more effectual
to place our faith where faith should reasonably be anchored, in God?

What else *is* the power that heals if it is not wholly
faith? The same faith that dispels a worry or some uncertainty dissolves a bodily affliction. Faith, whatever its mission, is directed *from, to,* and *within* the mind, never outside of it. There can be *nothing* outside of mind. Nor is it
in part that faith enters the picture, but rather does she
take over the *complete* business of restoring health to the
invalid, or tranquillity to the anxious heart.

Pray, then, when will mankind awake to this divine
truth which literally begs acceptance?

We are told in Luke:

"A woman having an issue of blood twelve years, which
had spent all her living upon physicians, neither could be
healed of any, came behind Jesus, and touched the border
of his garment: and immediately her issue of blood
stanched. . . . She declared unto him before all the people
for what cause she had touched him, and how she was
healed immediately. And Jesus said unto her, Daughter,
be of good comfort: thy faith hath made thee whole."

There lies the whole secret of healing, of overcoming
any obstacle, of living happily—the measure of your *faith.*
Jesus did not give this diseased woman a physical exam-

ination, nor did he give her drugs. He desired neither laboratory tests nor her genealogical history. There was no pretense for affect. There was no necessity for it, seeing that there was no fee to collect. He made it plain to her, as he did to all posterity, that her *faith* had made her whole. It was that simple. Truth is ever simple.

Should it not be concluded then, if we are to profit from the Master's remark to this woman, that the entire process of recovery is incumbent on faith in God alone?

To what avail are his teachings and demonstrations of healing if we are not to employ them to the advantage for which they were revealed to us?

Expecting to find health in a nauseous drug, rather than in God's power and wisdom, is the height of idolatry.

Dr. Oliver Wendell Holmes was particularly aware of this blind trust in drugs when he declared:

> "A silversmith will, for a dollar, make a small hoe, of solid silver, which will last for centuries, and will give a patient more comfort, if used for the removal of the accumulated epithelium and fungus growth which constitute the *fur* (on the tongue), than many a prescription with a splitfooted ℞ before it, addressed to the parts out of reach."

Even Claudius Galen, the Greek physician-philosopher, to whose memory the medical profession still pays homage after eighteen hundred years, was morally obliged to acknowledge the all-powerful influence of faith. He said, in these simple words:

> "Confidence and hope do *more* good than physic."

It is obvious that Galen did not imply that your confidence and hope in this instance be in your physician, but rather in yourself; for it is in your own self that the king-dom of God resides. The supreme power that is His actu-ally is at your finger tips to express and enjoy. It is a mock-ery of divine wisdom to believe that drugs and the scalpel have power to heal.

It is not that the medical profession is unaware of the mind playing an important role, if not the whole of it, in therapeutics; for the truth of the matter is it can no longer circumvent the fact that it is *completely* dependent upon mind. Nor is it any longer a secret that those sitting in high places of materia medica are increasingly aware of the layman being drawn to the sound logic of the mind's true power, thereby depriving a virtual industry of its livelihood.

That this is not a probability to be taken lightly, the medical fraternity has only recently sprouted an offshoot to its rapidly expanding province called psychosomatic medi-cine. This error, though somewhat more acceptable in nomenclature than the more unpleasant designation of psychiatry, was launched for the express purpose of com-bating the growing influence of metaphysical truth.

Psychosomatic medicine endeavors to unite the mind and material body into a single unit, or physical organism, which is not only a human or divine impossibility but the utter denial of truth. It would have you believe that bodily disorders can be induced by mental and emotional dis-turbances, a result of the interaction and interdependence of psychic and somatic phenomena.

Here psychosomatic medicine agrees with metaphysics in that bodily disorders are induced by mental distur-bances, and then it entangles itself inextricably in a maze of faulty speculation by claiming mind and matter to be in rapport. This it must do to uphold the vulnerable structure of materia medica. The microbe, in this instance, is left entirely out of the picture, unless it is proposed to be specially created through this relationship by illusion, as is the whole tapestry of its error.

The psyche, according to every lexicographer, is the spirit, mind, soul or mentality as distinguished from the physical and physiological.

Paul made it quite clear that the spiritual, or mental, cannot be united with a fleshly body into a single unit, or organism. The reason for this is plain: there being *no* physical body actually to unite. All is mind, and your physical body obviously can be nothing more than a conscious, though erroneous, image of thought.

This, the apostle corroborates:

> **"Ye are *not* in the flesh, but in the Spirit. . . . They which are the children of the flesh, these are *not* the children of God."**

What then are these children of the flesh?

A mistaken image of thought, an illusion, a misapprehension of the image of God.

How else then but by quackery, if we are to accept Paul's statement as authoritative, is it possible for any doctor to reach your complaint with a material drug? Or with a scalpel for that matter?

Ask yourself, in the depths of your consciousness: just how far is materia medica removed from the superstitions of the tribal medicine-man?

There can be but one answer: both are identical in fallacy, the former being learned charlatanism, the latter unlettered exorcism.

Wishing also to get a cut of the psychosomatic pie are the large pharmaceutical houses. As an example, Parke, Davis & Company of Detroit placed a full page advertisement in the *Saturday Evening Post* graphically portraying five masks in color, each representing anger, fear, jealousy, anxiety and worry.

The text read:

"Everyone knows that these and other disturbing emotions can play havoc with our mental poise. But not everyone realizes that such emotional disturbances can also make us physically ill. For we can actually worry ourselves into stomach ulcers, high blood pressure, allergies, and other disorders. And, of course, if we already have any of these disorders, nervous distress can make them worse.

"So if you find yourself, or any member of your family, becoming overburdened by emotional problems, or fearful of physical ills, do not drift along and try to cope with these problems alone. The wise thing to do is to see your doctor.

"It may surprise you to know how many of your physician's patients come to him with the same emotional burdens, how much he understands and sympathizes with such problems—and how wisely he can counsel you on the true causes of your condition, and the best remedial measures to take for your physical and mental well-being."

This clear admission that the mind provokes the physical body to become sick but is incapable of reversing the process is the paradox which makes the profession of medicine the satellite of the pharmaceutical houses.

You yourself must take inventory of the mental disturbances, or erroneous thoughts, that have brought you stomach ulcers, high blood pressure, allergies and other disorders, as enumerated by Parke, Davis & Co., and cast them out of your consciousness mentally. Indeed, the doctor can do nothing for you. Only *you* can do this. You must see the truth of your error, and then *unsee* it to get rid of it. This is changing your thought.

Paul puts it this way:

"Be ye transformed by the renewing of your mind."

The doctor's business is to drug you, and drug you he will, else you will not feel that he has done right by you, by his conscience, and by his profession. He unquestionably will prescribe a medicine for any one of the aforesaid disorders, simply because his alma mater had inculcated him with this procedure. And so it is that Parke, Davis & Company, as do all the other pharmaceutical manufacturers, come in for a cut of the psychosomatic pie.

Think of the mountains and rivers of medicinal preparations that have poured out of these factories around the world and into human stomachs since Hippocrates dignified the remedial prescription with his name! Yet, virtually every one of them has been discarded as ineffectual with the formulation of a new concoction to take its place. Today the fermentation of fungus has made obsolete yesterday's herb extracts, and tomorrow chemicals and atomic derivatives will likely supplant fungus rot. It has ever been so since humanity first sought a panacea in matter.

Dr. Flanders Dunbar, noted New York and Greenwich psychiatrist, and author of a book on psychosomatic medicine, maintains that, from medical studies available, eighty per cent of our population is in need of the services of a psychiatrist.

This incredible figure does not merely prove the potential commercial aspects of this latest field in medicine, but it rather makes mankind wonder what sort of blunder God had wrought upon the human race.

Of course if you are one to believe Dr. Dunbar, and believe it hard enough, you will outline this belief eventually in your consciousness to the extent that it will objectify exactly what you had outlined, and as a result you undoubtedly will be a regular visitor soon to a psychiatrist's office. This is the subtle way of propagating disease.

If you would heal your sick body, you must, as Paul had pointed out,

"be transformed by the renewing of your mind."

This transformation is knowing that God never made an imperfect man. It is therefore obvious that Dr. Dunbar, like all psychiatrists, is wrestling with an illusion no less than the patient who believes he can be healed with psychosomatic medicine, the same old nauseous nostrum put up in a newly-designed package. Little wonder that the public recoils from psychiatry, as it will from psychosomatic medicine when the truth of being is fairly understood.

Frequently it takes a good part of a lifetime as a medical practitioner to be convinced, as was Dr. William S. Sadler, that the drugging and cutting up of the body is not the answer to man's afflictions. After prolonged observation, this well-known and respected professor of physiologic therapeutics concluded:

"For centuries it has been known that mind could influence matter. . . . Indeed, the higher we ascend in the level of consciousness, the less sensation we have, and the more appreciation we have of the real meaning of things. . . .

Human health and happiness cannot be greatly promoted if the civilized races do not bear in mind two great truths: first, the influence of the mind in the prevention of disease; second, the marvelous power of Nature (also the mind) to heal."

Dr. Sadler has grasped no small part, if not the full import, of pure metaphysics. Again the mind has been enthroned with the nobility it deserves by another schooled in the dogma of medicine. It is without saying, this spiritually-minded physician has tasted of the divine elixir through realization of the great truth which he has uttered:

"The higher we ascend in the level of consciousness, the less sensation we have, and the more appreciation we have of the real meaning of things."

It is well to consider here the above shred of wisdom in contrast with a spoonful of unpalatable medicine concocted in ignorance, if only to learn that without benefit of the mind, consciousness, the unknowing spoonful of medicine could have no more substance, identity, action, nor purpose, than the inside of a vacuum.

CHAPTER X

MIND IS the only power. There is none other. Too, mind is the only substance and identity. It is the substance of your body, as well as its identity. Moreover, mind is the substance and identity of everything, your friends, possessions, automobile, ambitions—yes, of the entire universe. All that has been conceived and created is part and parcel of the kingdom of God, and this complete kingdom is *within* you, your mind.

This kingdom *cannot* be in any material body for the simple reason that there is no material body for it to be in. Nor can this kingdom be in a *belief* of a material body, inasmuch as this would admit of reality dwelling in nonexistence.

Everything that God has made is wholly mental in conception, in its evolvement, and its unfoldment. And, more, all of it exists eternally within His mind. We merely are the reflection of it, that is we apprehend creation through conscious receptivity. There is *no* other thing existent, much less matter.

This accords with what St. John had said:

"All things were made by Him; and without Him was not anything made that was made."

Matter therefore must be an erroneous belief, being made, as it was, without Him. Nothing can be added to His creation, except it be a human *belief* of something.

Your true substance and identity are mental, and this is the *only* constitution which your body has. Being a spiritual body, it is a three-dimensional idea, or image, made from the substance of God's thought, having been conceived in, sustained in, and forever abides in, His mind, as does everything else which He has created. Although this body *appears* to your erring sense of things to be constructed from matter, and consequently physical, it is none the less a purely mental manifestation.

To repeat again, what Paul had stated,

"Ye are *not* in the flesh, but in the Spirit,"

is but another way of telling you that your real, and only, body is a conscious picture in your mind, and this picture is the reflection or image of God. Incidentally, all things, or ideas, that He had created—including yourself—is in His mind. If we did not live in God's consciousness we could not be aware of His other ideas. The mistaken belief that this mental image of your body is physical, engenders the kindred errors of disease and inharmony that are peculiar to this distorted picture in your thought.

Mentally seeing, as well as feeling, the truth that the body is in mind, rather than the mind in body, begins at once to set you free from the claims of disease and discord. This higher level of consciousness opens a new vista to your understanding, as Dr. Sadler had pointed out, and your appreciation of the real meaning of things becomes increasingly greater.

The loom that ceaselessly weaves the pattern of spiritual

existence upon the screen of your consciousness is the Creator who made heaven and earth. You are the warp and weft of that pattern, and as perfect and eternal as its design.

Indeed, the years do not enfeeble man. Years, like inches and feet, or minutes and hours, are merely measuring devices in which man imprisons himself. Years have no power to make old, decrepit or impotent, nor do they have any such knowledge of itself. It is solely man's thinking that makes him senile, submitting himself voluntarily as he does to the physical limitations of time. He literally measures out his own destiny with a calendar and his self-inflicted infirmities. Eternality alone is real, and everlastingly reminds us that man is spiritual by keeping alive in him the spark of hope and faith.

When Jesus stated, emphatically,

"Let man deny himself,"

he was specifically alluding to the so-called material body. The Master's very phraseology made it plain that the physical form was not man, God's image and likeness. Certainly he could not have meant, by any stretch of the imagination, that you deny your spiritual heritage; for such a denial would not only be absurd, but would deprive man of his entity entirely.

Your body shall ever be an enigma to you so long as you assume it to be of physical composition rather than a conscious picture within your own mind. Realizing, with solid conviction, that everything is mental, your mind and body become inseparably *one*, since both are of the same substance. Choosing to believe otherwise, that your body is the substance of material flesh, is to invite all the discords that are subject to this belief of flesh.

When you fairly see that mind is the only substance and identity, your true body will appear to you on the mirror of your consciousness much as a motion picture is projected on the screen in a theatre. This conscious reflection is God's image and likeness, with which His kingdom is correlated; and this is the truth which Jesus said you shall know, and which, as a result of your knowing, shall make you free.

Paul put it this way:

"Look not at the things which are seen, but at the things which are not seen: for the things which are seen are temporal (illusory); but the things which are not seen are eternal (real)."

In this revelation by the apostle he is plainly stating that that which appears physical, or temporal (illusory), to you is not real, and therefore to disregard it as such; while that which is unfolded spiritually within your consciousness is the reality which you actually have been experiencing all the time, but mistakenly believed to be physical. This spiritual unfoldment has the divine stamp of God's creation; and, hence, it is everlasting.

That which your erring sense believes physical is similarly an image of thought, not outside of your mind, nor around it, which you seem to think, but *in* it. This is the temporal illusion, or erroneous picture of the spiritual, at which Paul said not to look.

You undoubtedly will ask, and rightly so: what does all this prove, that man and the creation are *not* material, and the kingdom of God is within us?

It proves just this: by understanding and practicing the truth of being, we can individually demonstrate all that Jesus had taught us, the complete mastery over disease, adversity, poverty, unhappiness, and even the power over death.

When you have reasonably acquired this understanding, you will have *all* that your heart could possibly desire.

Need there be more?

Again, it may be asked: what difference is there in seeing something that God had made, which is real, and seeing the same thing before my conscious vision when it does not actually appear?

You see the sun by day, actually, but at night the same sun that you see in your conscious vision is simply a *recollection* of the real one that you had seen during the day. If there were no such thing as a sun created by God, you could never have a conscious vision of it in recollection, nor otherwise, since there would be *nothing* suggestive of that idea to conceive or recollect. Indeed, recollection is not error, but rather is error seeing something which is contrary to the real in substance. Recollection, like the sun, also is God's idea.

Believing that the sun is matter is error. And to believe that you can profit by stealing, concealing, sharp dealing, or by any other form of duplicity, when God, alone, supplies us with all our needs, is likewise error. Little does one know the might and omnipotence of *mind* who would gain by dishonesty, or a mercenary heart.

Said Marcus Aurelius:

"The mind, unmastered by the passions, is a very citadel, for a man has no fortress more impregnable wherein to find refuge."

This wise philosopher had penetrated the illusory barriers of matter to learn that the only power and reality existent lie within individual man himself. Within the refuge of his mind is *all* that God had created.

All that appears to be *outside* of your body, the stars, trees, your home, the soaring eagle, actually is within your consciousness. The belief that *you* are material gives all else the illusion of appearing material also. All that is outside of you is merely projected so in your thought. This, obviously, is the situation with disease on your body. Were disease real, it would be impossible to be removed therefrom.

Dr. Howard Wilcox Haggard, Professor at Yale, in his contribution to the *Story of Human Error,* said:

> "The mind influences the action of the body. . . . The lame have thrown away their crutches, the halt have walked, the blind have seen. Similar miracles have been performed with . . . treatment that catches and holds the attention and inspires belief in recovery."

It makes no difference what the affliction might be, whether acute or chronic, deep-seated or inherited, it must imperatively dissolve before mind when the error which holds it fast is removed.

There is no substitute for metaphysical treatment. *All* is mind, and *in* mind. There is no matter whatever, only a belief of it.

Because you are unable at once to demonstrate the truths herein, it does not imply that they are not demonstrable. The fact that Jesus demonstrated them and assured us that we, too, can do likewise, and *more*—as the widespread evidence of it is being revealed daily—should be sufficient warrant that they can be successfully manifested.

You need only to practice truth's rule, as you would expect to do in any scientific endeavor. The countless people today that are demonstrating these truths to a degree commensurable with their understanding is ample proof of the verity of the Master's teachings.

Thought is the *only* power and identity; all else is merely illusion.

It is generally believed that man invents, or creates, unusual mechanisms such as the combustion engine, dynamo, television, phonograph, and the like, when in reality he only *discovers* these ideas of God which are reflected to his consciousness. Inventions are not creations, for God alone creates. Man simply becomes aware of what He already has conceived.

Man can neither invent nor discover anything which God has not already created, for nothing exists out of which to invent or discover excepting those things which He alone has brought forth in consciousness. That this is so, Jesus unmistakably confirms:

"The Son can do nothing of himself, but what he seeth the Father do: for what things soever He doeth, these also doeth the Son likewise."

There is absolutely nothing that you can conceive, invent or produce, unless you fabricate it from God's multitudinous thoughts, which are the ideas you discover in your consciousness. This is utilizing the unfolding kingdom that is within you.

Think not that what you look out upon is separate in substance or being from yourself. This is an error of matter. Everything that you see, hear, feel, taste and smell is in yourself.

Sir Isaac Newton, discoverer of the law of gravitation, had a vague idea of the profundity of the infinite, when he said:

> "I do not know what I may appear to the world, but to myself I seem to have been only a boy playing on the seashore and diverting myself in finding a smoother pebble or a prettier shell than ordinary, while the great ocean of truth lay all undiscovered before me."

Diseased thinking makes a diseased body as surely as thought gives impulse to action. When a condition of disorder becomes first evident, your erroneous thought instantly calls up fear to worsen this very situation which you yourself have unwittingly induced. And unless you begin promptly to reverse your thinking in the same order, you will inexorably play out the whole diapason of material existence to its final note, death itself.

Thoughts are things, and the act of thinking is much like newly-poured cement in its consistency. If it be a harmful thought, it can be changed more readily in its primary state, similarly to altering the consistency of the cement; but once this thought sets into conviction, like the hardening of mortar, it requires a proportionally greater understanding of the laws of being to resolve.

As the plant springs forth from its seed, so every act, experience and accomplishment of man springs from the seeds of his thought. The human mind, in this respect, is not unlike a garden. Let him sow good seed into its soil, and as sure as the sun rises in the East will beautiful experiences, like lovely flowers, come forth to enrich his life.

But let him sow a poor quality of seed in this same soil, and a monotonous existence, not unlike the grim aspect of barren land, will be his lot.

Dr. George W. Crile well knew the philosophy of this inescapable truth from his practical experience and observation as a physician, surgeon, and teacher of materia medica. Said he:

> "Man has conquered everything but himself . . . He hates and fears . . . and in these emotions and strivings are laid the foundations of many diseases. The effect of fear, grief, worry and jealousy on the physical body is seen in the changes in the cells of the brain, the adrenals and the liver, and in the numerous diseases and disabilities."

If what Dr. Crile has said is true, and here he is in absolute accord with metaphysics as to the exciting cause of disease, why should not the mind reasonably be the *antidote* also for what is contended mind has brought into existence. It is obvious where hate has induced disease, man's common intelligence should tell him that his hatred must first be removed if he would dissolve the disease. This is the high point of Jesus' teachings, his compelling commandment to *love* one another.

Still materia medica would dissolve these externalized evidences of hatred, fear, grief, worry, jealousy, and the whole range of evil thinking, with non-intelligent matter, or cut them out with a knife.

That disease is not induced by microbes and germs floating through the air, but by fear and hate and envy, and the like, the Master substantiated, when he said to the impotent man whom he had healed:

> "Sin no more, lest a worse thing come unto thee."

As for microbes and germs and contagion being the source of disease, as humankind is led to believe by the medical fraternities, Jesus emphatically declared:

> **"There is nothing from without a man, that entering into him can defile him: but the things which come out of him."**

Fear, hate and envy, to enumerate but a few evils, are the exciting sins that provoke disease. Anger is a deadly poison. Only when man learns to subdue his passions will he discover that his body has correspondingly become immune to disease and discord.

Professor Elmer Gates, of the Smithsonian Institution, and Director of the Laboratory of Psychology and Psychurgy, in Washington, D. C., in his scientific reports of experiments on the emotional effects of the mind, corroborates the conclusions of Dr. Crile with this interesting account:

> **"When the breath of a patient was passed through a tube cooled with ice so as to condense the volatile qualities of the respiration, the iodide of rhodopsin, mingled with these condensed products, produced no observable precipitate. But, within five minutes after the patient became angry, there appeared a brownish precipitate, which indicates the presence of a chemical compound produced by the emotion. This compound, extracted and administered to men and animals, caused stimulation and excitement. Extreme sorrow, such as mourning for the loss of a child recently deceased, produced a gray precipitate; remorse a pink precipitate, etc. My experiments show the irascible, malevolent, and depressing emotions generate in the system injurious compounds, some of which are extremely poisonous; also, that agreeable happy emotions**

generate chemical compounds of nutritious value, which stimulate the cells that manufacture energy . . . My experiments have demonstrated that every emotion of a false and disagreeable nature produces a poison in the blood and cell tissues. These poisons affect the health of the germ-cells."

It is well to remind yourself frequently that thoughts which produce pleasant and kindly smiles and that good all-over-feeling also produce, when turned to evil speculations, poison, disease and invalidism.

Many years ago the staid British Medical Journal made this significant observation on the supremacy of mind:

"Disease of the body is so much influenced by the mind that in each case we have to understand the patient quite as much as the malady."

The medical fraternity, hard pressed by the revealing power of truth, is becoming more and more aware that the incubus of disease has its inception in the mind. But here the practicing profession is confronted with a most perplexing question: under what method of treatment should this uncompromising intruder submit?

Obviously, the mind can never be reached with materia medica; and to yield to the simple expedient of *truth*, as practiced by the Master and his followers, is to allow a highly remunerative vocation crumble under the weight of its own fallacy.

And so it became desirable to launch psychosomatic medicine amidst the fanfare of medical progress. This it would introduce into the mental bloodstream of human gullibility. Only the future can adequately determine the evil of its present-day experimentations.

Not all within the fold of the medical profession adhere to the so-called ethics imposed on that body by the political oligarchs of the American Medical Association. Dr. Frederick Peterson, reputable New York neurologist, was but one of many practitioners that saw the reality of things in contrast with their material appearance. He declared:

> "Matter has vanished into something unsubstantial, and becomes an illusion . . . If we cut a certain worm in two, one part grows a head and the other a tail. Some lizards grow a tail in the place of one lost . . . Certain crawfish will grow one of their complicated legs in the place of one amputated. These extraordinary healing processes are more than simple chemistry . . . Injury to any part of the human body stimulates the chemistry of the whole body, and starts a rush of repairing cells to the seat of injury. This is the *healing power of Nature,* which has been for two thousand years a special shibboleth to physicians . . . It seems to me that some great organized effort should be made to study the mind in relation to the body . . . There is abundant evidence that the mind, particularly the emotions, affects physical functions of all kinds."

One need only weigh intelligently the logic of Dr. Peterson's graphic observation to see the abysmal ignorance claiming to assist the divine forces (Nature) in her work. If God's wisdom and substance created man, surely this same omnipotence must possess the means to sustain him in perfect health.

If growth and healing come naturally to lower forms of life, why should man expect less for himself from the Almighty?

To quote Dr. William S. Sadler once more:

"It seems almost impossible to convince many people that
... health and disease are largely matters of sowing and
reaping, and that health or disease is determined by certain fixed mental and physical laws."

Health is *ever* a mental law, spiritual law, while disease
is an affinity of physical illusion. There can be no perfection in physical law, since physical law is an erroneous belief. Such law always has been an error from time immemorial. Perfection lies only in God's spiritual law, and this
is the only law that actually exists. Any other law is but a
mistaken sense of spiritual law, and it is in this mistaken
sense alone that disease exerts its influence.

All the physical organs of man are imperfect from the
very nature of their unreality, seeing that all physical phenomena merely is an illusory conception of everything
spiritually substantial.

The famous scientist and physiologist, Baron Von Helmholtz, whose lifetime of study in physiological optics had
richly contributed to the present-day knowledge of oph-
thalmology, gives this bit of interesting information about
material phenomena:

"If an optician would sell me an instrument which had all
the defects of the human eye, I should think myself quite
justified in blaming his carelessness in the strongest
terms, and giving him back his instrument."

What God has made is eternally perfect. What appears
to human sense as matter, man's body for example, is always
susceptible to discord and decay. This is so because what
is believed to be physical is merely a misapprehension of
its true counterpart, spiritual reality. Such is the fact

whether it be a material eye, as Baron Von Helmholtz has specifically depicted, or any human organ or thing that is believed to be constituted of matter.

A friend of the author, a high school teacher, had become stone-blind and destined never to see again by several outstanding eye specialists. This prognostic consensus was arrived at only after every possible avenue of skill and knowledge, based on materia medica, was exhausted. The optic nerves had completely atrophied, and a crystallization from hemorrhage had formed solidly under the corneas.

One day, during this dark interval in her life, as she lay crushed by this tragedy, she was urged to turn to God for a healing, as so few do when all material means have been expended.

In an endeavor to lift her spirit, two passages from the Scriptures were read to her:

"God is our refuge and strength, a very present help in trouble . . . With men this is impossible; but with God *all* things are possible."

With the same profound and absorbing faith that drew to the Master the blind, the dumb and the halt, she, too, was gently drawn to that spiritual fountainhead of truth which he symbolized. With a minimum of metaphysical instruction, based solely on the simple teachings of Jesus and Paul, among others, that man is transformed by the *renewing* of his mind, she began to grasp the grand reality of being, and saw that nothing God had made—including her sight—could be harmed, much less destroyed.

Her healing, as a result, was quickly attained, and without the usual discomforts and period of convalescence. It was a complete healing, to the astonishment of the several specialists who had attended her, while at the same time her eyes took on an added lustre and even better vision than at any time prior to her affliction.

Here was a demonstration of healing precisely as Jesus said you were capable of effecting. Neither scalpel nor medication was employed. It was wholly a manifestation of mind. The belief of atrophied optic nerves and crystallization from hemorrhage under the corneas disappeared in the degree that she saw the truth that man is not material but spiritual. Nothing real disappeared, only an illusion.

Jakob Boehme, the renowned shoemaker of Gorlitz, Germany, who had the rare experience of divine illumination, saw in his mind what comparatively few men have been privileged to see. He said:

"If you will behold your own self and the outer world, and what is taking place therein, you will find that you, with regard to your external being, are that external world."

This well-known and generally-recognized mystic was stating, in his simple tongue, what Jesus had long declared:

"The kingdom of God is within you."

Your real self, not the spurious counterfeit appearing as matter, is the image of God; and His kingdom *is* this image.

Only by silently beholding, realizing in your consciousness, the profundity, grandeur and perfection of the spiritual world, can you enter into it. This world is entirely within yourself, within your mind. So is the illusion called the physical, or material, world which appears outside of yourself. Beholding this physical picture in your consciousness, you unavoidably reap that of which you believe yourself a part.

Displaying an ill-humored countenance is revealing the naked thought of irritability which you have given birth and unfoldment in your consciousness. A sour stomach, or a rebellious one, is merely mirroring the quality of your thinking. This is equally true whether your complaint is an ailing kidney, a troublesome heart, or a malignant tumor.

Anger and resentment are readily observed in one's facial expression by their intensity of emotion, such as stormy eyes, tightened muscles, clenched teeth and blanched face. This you can easily discern in another, inasmuch as they are observable externally; but just what do you determine must be taking place, because of this intensity of emotion, in the *inner* parts of this person, his heart, lungs, liver, glands, and other vitals?

No less than the distorted phenomenon on his face is the distortion in his thought, repeating itself in every organ and activity within the physical body. All of it is in his mind, including his physical body.

Here, then, is the exciting cause of all disorder, one's evil propensities, such as hatred, malice, revenge, envy, and the like. They poison the blood stream, obstruct the secretions, impede the complex functions of the nervous system. Wrong thinking ties the intestines in seeming knots, causes food to lie like stones in the stomach, brings on headaches, dizzy spells, aches and pains, and the innumerable other discomforts and afflictions peculiar to ill health.

Love alone is their antidote.

If one would promote his state of health, he would do well to learn from Booker T. Washington, who said:

"I will allow no man to drag me down so low as to make me hate him."

No one, understanding God, can really love Him and yet hate his fellow man. This famous Negro educator was wiser by far, and more spiritually-minded, than any of his oppressors.

To hate *anyone* is dense ignorance, while harboring the spirit of vindictiveness is stooping to the selfsame level of the one to whom you would return evil.

Marcus Antoninus sagely said:

"The best sort of revenge is not to be like him who did the injury."

You clothe yourself with the garments spun from your own thoughts as surely as you obey the impulses which spring from the same source.

Spiritual law cannot be circumvented. Love is God's design. To inject the human element of evil into this design is the height of folly. Its fruits invariably are disease, want and woe.

Paul brings out this point clearly:

"Be not deceived; God is not mocked: for whatsoever a man soweth, that shall he also reap."

The next tragic step taken by man, after he has experienced the first symptoms of disorder, is to believe in its reality; for here, unwittingly, he mentally develops its pathological progress to the point where it externalizes itself as morbid disease on his physical body. Frightened by his own enveloping thoughts, he digs deeper still into his inexhaustible reserve of error, and comes up with an ogre to which he himself gives all its assumed power, and this he identifies as *fear*.

Obviously, the morbid condition at once evolves itself deeper yet in its own morbidity, and sooner or later he discovers himself headed for a fatal turn in his illness unless a countering thought takes possession meanwhile of his mind. This latter thought which he calls up in himself, if indeed he does, is a *faith* either in the power of God to reverse the course of the disease or in materia medica. If the balance of this faith should fall short of overcoming the extent of the involvement, he will have enacted the entire drama, even unto death, which he alone has directed on the stage of his consciousness.

It is because man believes that he exists separately from God, at least as a material entity, that he fears his own thoughts. Surely there is nothing else to fear, for God made everything good, and that which was made without Him is illusion, or erroneous belief. Were man thoroughly aware that he is *one* with God, spiritually coexistent with Him in His mind, he would never fear anything.

Dr. Henry Maudsley, Fellow of the Royal College of Physicians, and Professor of Medical Jurisprudence at University College in London, said:

> "To me it seems not unreasonable to suppose that the mind may stamp its tone, if not its very features, on the individual elements of the body, inspiring them with hope and energy, or inflicting them with despair or feebleness."

Fear is the sustenance on which materia medica thrives. That which brings cold beads of sweat to the brow or perspiration rolling from the palms of your hands is the same terror that produces death.

Indeed, little is known of the emotional tendencies and reactions of the mind when callous, and frequently venal, practitioners deliberately frighten credulous patients into submitting to certain forms of operative treatment where even a child would sense ultimate disaster.

Dr. Max Thorek was neither blind to such practices nor insensible to the way the mere suggestion of surgery acts upon the constitutional and functional processes of the body. He declared:

"Fatalities are too numerous to recite where in anticipation of operation patients have died from fear."

Here is something to think about: is the mind, the only substance and identity of man, forever to be thrust aside in deference to an illusory body?

The famed Dr. Grantly Dick Read, internationally-known obstetrician, dared publicly to expose through his widely-read book, *Childbirth Without Fear,* and condensed in Reader's Digest, the incredible fallacies under which a supposedly enlightened medical profession is practicing. He said:

"Childbirth is a primitive function intended by Nature to be painless. . . . The more cultured the races of man have become, the more dogmatic have they been in pronouncing childbirth to be a painful and dangerous ordeal. . . . If a woman's mind, conditioned since childhood by gossip and mythology, interprets the new sensations caused by the first contractions as pain, the fancied and expected pain results in fear. And the fear results in muscular tension. . . . Therefore, fear, pain and tension are the three

evils which are not normal to the natural design, but have been introduced in the course of civilization. If fear, pain and tension go hand in hand, then it must be possible to eliminate pain by relieving tension and overcoming fear. . . . It is impossible to protect women from fear of childbirth if they are ignorant of the truth. . . . Obstetricians have been educated to believe that all labors are painful. They have made a routine of using analgesic or anesthetic. . . . How long, oh, how long will this nonsense go on? Can the scientific mind see no further than drugs and anesthetics? We know death occurs from the use of these things; harm to both mother and child is recorded by a large number of competent observers. . . . Surely it is safer to introduce a mental process than a dangerous drug. The best, and safest, anesthetic is a controlled and educated mind."

Many maternity hospitals have proven the verity of Dr. Read's exposure; and where intelligent women have shown a desire to *unlearn* the errors and fables handed down to them from childhood, they have been delivered of their babies without anxiety or discomfort. God is a merciful Creator, and it is inane to believe that He made woman to suffer in childbirth in order to fulfil His design.

The same fear that produces muscular tension in childbirth provokes similar disturbances in all of the body's organs and functions. It freezes the blood that has been flowing gently through the veins, paralyzes locomotion, makes faint the heart, pales the cheeks, upsets the stomach. Fear starts the wheels of chemistry in the body to produce toxemia, which in turn makes sluggish the bowels, dulls the eyes, sallows the complexion.

Fear is merely a thought, a rabid one to be sure, set loose

in your consciousness much as a threatening dog is turned out to run amuck children at play. Unless it is promptly cast out of your mind, as you would cast out any evil, it will become your master.

You give fear its nativity, nurture it, gratify its demands, and when at last it takes on proportions beyond your control, you stand trembling in awe before it. Moreover, you seek protection from it, from its terror, protection from your own thoughts.

In consequence, if it be a bodily disorder, you call a doctor. The medicinal balm which he prescribes and which allays your fear, if indeed it does, is your own thought. And this thought, which annuls the fear, is the same thought that gave the fear its power in the first place. It should therefore be plain that the power which conceived the monster is equally capable of dissolving it. This is done solely by knowing the truth of its unreality.

The brilliant thinker, Goethe, said:

> **"Fear is a condition of sloth in which any enemy may take possession of us."**

This condition of sloth, as pointed out by the German poet, is the familiar disinclination on the part of man to understand the inner power, or the kingdom of God that is within him. Hence, his lack of cooperation with himself to dispel the ills which he alone has originated. Obviously, it is far more desirable to surrender himself to indolence and materia medica and be carried along with the current of illusion.

It is little wonder that darkness rules the minds of men.

Ralph Waldo Emerson, during the Civil War, visited the Springfield arsenal. After viewing the great stock-piles of munitions, small compared to present-day standards, he said:

"At first I was struck with fear at all this panoply of war, until I recalled that it all arose out of a thought, and a thought can melt it away."

This was true nearly a hundred years ago, and it still is true today. It was true a thousand years ago, five thousand years ago, yes—since the dawn of creation, and it shall *ever* be true so long as God's kingdom is designed such as it is.

"A *thought* can melt it away!"

Indeed, nothing else can.

So does thought melt disease away, in fact *any* inharmony. Medicine and the scalpel have never removed anything, not so much as an illusion, for mind must remove even this.

Your consciousness is the kingdom which God has created. You have scarcely begun to scratch the surface of its infinite possibilities. To regard the dominion of your mind lightly is utter sin. In the degree that you do so, you expose a comparable ignorance.

Nothing of a physical nature can withstand the invincible powers of the mind. The most formidable barriers, the greatest masses of matter, the remotest recesses within the earth, are all conquered by it. *Everything* must yield to mind. The very heavens are laid open to it.

The well-meaning physician, the anxious patient submitting to him, and a trusting public that shares the credulity of both, are assuredly lost in darkness if they entertain the slightest belief that power of any kind can be dispensed from vials of loathsome extracts in the back room of a drug store. This is hardly a step in human progress, if progress it may be, over the incantations and exorcisms practiced among the pagans.

Dr. George W. Crile, searching scientifically into the labyrinths of disease, its remedies and preventives, learned this startling fact, which in turn he passed on to posterity:

"One of the mysteries of the human race is the fact that civilized man is subject to certain diseases that *rarely* attacked primitive man and never appear in wild animals. These are various nervous and mental disorders, goiter, asthenia, Raynaud's disease, diabetes, peptic ulcer, hypertension and coronary disease."

Why is this so?

Dr. Crile gives the obvious answer. This outstanding pillar in the faculty of modern medicine, drawing upon his researches in the life and habits of the undomesticated beasts, added:

"Unlike man, wild animals do not appear to think about themselves; therefore they do not think in error about themselves."

And so it was with primitive man, to a greater extent than is generally suspected.

There you have the seed, root and flower of all disease and disorder, thinking in error. Man has gradually retrograded in health and longevity in the ratio that he has departed from the truth, the primitive laws of God, and indoctrinated himself in the fallacies of materialism.

The stamina and virility of the antediluvians tell us, if nothing else, that the human race has lost its way somewhere in the wilderness of physical knowledge. In short, whereas primitive man has been guided more or less by divine intuition, modern man is influenced almost entirely by the errors of a mortal intellect.

Modern man has resorted to every vagary of material invention in an endeavor to recapture his lost health, and there is no reason to believe that he shall not continue to do so until the hand of death claims him, unless he awakens meanwhile and learns that health and disease are merely states of mind. His sick thought must be instructed in divine wisdom and understanding to respond to health, as it has long been schooled in materialism to provoke disease.

If a diseased man's faith in a rabbit's foot or other such fetish to restore health is greater than in the unsavory mixture of a pharmacist's concoction, the noisome concoction will be far more profitably used in turning lead into gold than in healing his complaint.

Claudius Galen well knew the power of thought even in his time; for the poet, Stefano Guazzo, some fourteen hundred years later, was constrained to gently refresh the human memory of that day, thus:

> **"Galen sayeth, 'the disquiet of the minde breedeth the disease of the bodye'; and that he hath cured many diseases by bringing the pulses into good temper, and by quieting the minde."**

Attempting to heal diseased matter with an extract of more matter, without reckoning mind as the sole factor in the whole process, is educated ignorance.

The Roman Stoic philosopher, Lucius Annaeus Seneca,

was aware of this truth even before Galen came into the world. Said he:

"The mind is the master over every kind of fortune; itself acts in both ways, being the cause of its own happiness and misery."

The many miracles of healing from Lourdes to Ste. Anne De Beaupre, together with those at tombstones scattered across every nation, under which lie decomposed bodies believed to possess power to bring divine blessings from the Creator, are nothing more than mere demonstrations of faith. They are a misdirected faith to be sure, but this misdirected faith proves beyond all question that the power revealed to heal them of their afflictions is within themselves rather than in the inanimate stone and wood shrines. The omnipotence of Almighty God can *never* be reached by, or through, these deified objects of matter.

Touching a hallowed stone, or being lowered into a pool of consecrated water, surely has no efficacy of itself to heal. The healing power is in the mind of the one benefited. This power is the divine kingdom that God forged and weaved into the image and likeness of Himself. When man fairly sees this truth, his healings will come readily wherever he might be. Inanimate shrines that draw man for any purpose other than curiosity smacks of the idolatry practiced in antiquity.

God's power is ever present within you. It constantly envelops and permeates you. It is exclusively a mental power, and always available in your consciousness, the only place power can express and manifest itself. This is the healing factor, and needs only to be *realized* in order to bring it into your experience.

This realization held *steadfastly* in thought, is availing yourself of spiritual power, putting it profitably to use. It is likewise bringing into conscious focus the image of God which you are. Moreover, it is evidencing your faith, which alone is the restorative agency that makes perfect. And, lastly, it is acknowledging the fact that everything exists and takes place in mind, since there is no such thing as matter anywhere.

All, *everything,* is your conscious reception of God's thinking, the apprehending of His ideas. This unfoldment in your mind is His kingdom, which always has been, and always will be, within *you.*

Strive to discover and become aware of the innumerable ideas in this kingdom. They are yours, every one. Such realization of God's infinitude within you is the only power there is. Drink deeply of it. Immerse yourself in its inspiration. Breathe it into every cell and corpuscle in your being. It is *all* a mental accomplishment.

Jesus confirmed the fact time and again that the power of healing, no less than the attainment of harmony over discord, belongs solely unto mind. He said, plainly:

"All things, whatsoever ye shall ask in prayer, believing, ye shall receive."

A brief examination of this passage should convince the most skeptical person that everything is *in,* and *of,* mind.

Where else, if not in mind, can you possibly receive any benefit from God in answer to your prayer?

That mind plays the leading, and *only,* role in the drama of existence, Dr. Frederick Peterson reveals from case histories of prominent European and American neurologists. To cite a few:

> "Baron Richard von Krafft-Ebing, noted German professor of neurology, placed a postage stamp on the arm of a young woman, telling her it was a fly-blister and would produce a blister in a few hours. She did not see what he had applied. He carefully bandaged and sealed the spot so that it could not be tampered with. The blister actually appeared in a few hours."

Here is a concrete example of a concept having birth, unfoldment and externalization in the space of a few hours. It not only was conceived and excited *in* mind, but its externalization entirely was *of* mind. Its physical appearance outside of mind was simply an illusion of material sense. There absolutely is *nothing* outside of mind.

Resuming Dr. Peterson's case histories:

> "Another internationally-known neurologist, Dr. Pierre Janet, Professor of Psychology, College of France, had a patient with a religious ecstasy who believed she was to receive the stigmata of Christ. A blet began to appear on each foot. He covered one foot with a bandage, a sheet of mica and a seal, and watched the development of an actual ulcer on each foot. They were precisely like those seen in the paintings and statues of the body of Christ."

This illustration of belief by Dr. Janet is virtually identical in its manifestation with that revealed by Dr. Krafft-Ebing.

Another case history related by Dr. Peterson is one with which almost every physician is familiar to some greater or lesser extent, even in his own experience:

> "Dr. Alexis Carrel saw a woman at Lourdes one summer who had a large indolent ulcer on her back for nine years, with unhealthy granulations which no ordinary

treatment with salves or escharotics had improved. Twelve
hours after the Lourdes ceremonies the granulations had
taken on a healthy appearance and the ulcer had dimin-
ished by several millimetres in diameter. He had seen and
measured the ulcer before and after the healing."

Here is incontrovertible proof that faith, working
through *mind,* is the absolute healer, and that materia
medica is an imposition on credulous humanity. The blind
faith that heals when touching a crumbling tombstone is
the same influencing agency that heals, if it does, when you
quaff a dose of disagreeable medicine.

These examples of causal action and phenomena are
what the brilliant physicist, Sir Arthur Stanley Eddington,
inferred, when he declared:

**"The mind may indeed be said to create its own physical
environment."**

Notwithstanding all evidence to the contrary, everything
that we are is the result of what we have thought. The
happiness of our lives, no less than our health and well-
being, depends solely upon the quality of thinking we
allow into our consciousness.

Edmund Spenser, English poet, in extolling the supremacy and influence of thought, said:

**"It is the mind that maketh good or evil, that maketh
wretch or happy, rich or poor."**

Whatever *good* we think and hold secure within the
sanctum of our minds, no matter how unimportant these
thoughts might be, externalizes itself in its rightful place
to the advantage of all mankind.

Peace of mind can be had in no other way than through

the processes of mind. To believe that you can profit through dishonesty, cunning, deceit, or any such wrongdoing, is to invite disaster sooner or later, for disease, discontent, and all the other inharmonies of mortal man, are the fruits of their corrupt seed. You cannot forever escape the judgment of justice. It is eternally weighing you and your deeds on the scales of your own consciousness.

This is made unusually clear by Philo Judaeus:

"The mind is the witness to each individual of the things which he has planned in secret, while conscience is an incorruptible judge and the most unerring of all judges."

Man has only *one* identity, and it is spiritual, or mental. That which appears otherwise, the physical counterpart, is a deception, and this false phenomenon is the error typified by Satan, or evil. Not realizing that the kingdom of God actually is *within* him, man naturally assumes that it exists *outside* of his material body. This kingdom, or creation, which he mistakenly sees outside of himself as being material, is merely an illusion within his own mind. He is projecting it outside of himself, in his own consciousness, as the story creation within the motion picture film is projected outside of itself, with the aid of light, on to the screen. Neither projection, as matter, is real, but illusion.

Jesus stressed the fact rather forcefully that the kingdom of God is *within* man, and this statement definitely admits of it being mental. The belief that the kingdom is material obviously compels man to project his conviction *outside* of himself, for simple logic precludes placing a physical kingdom *within* the outline of his material body, much less everyone else's body. It is therefore easily seen, in light of the Master's teachings, that thought alone is the composition of all physical phenomena.

Scientifically, you are God's thoughts—with a varying amount of your own thrust in to obscure the true picture—projected upon the screen of your consciousness.

Alfred Tennyson, poet laureate of England, had many times seen and felt this truth in his own experience. Said he:

> **"There are moments when the flesh is nothing to me. . . . The spiritual *is* the real; it belongs to one more than the hand and foot. You may tell me that my (material) hand and foot are only imaginary symbols of my existence. I could believe you, but you never, never can convince me that the *I* is not an eternal reality, and that the spiritual is not the true and real part of me."**

The *I,* which Lord Tennyson says is an eternal reality and the true part of himself, is the conscious image of God. This image is solely mental. It was the poet's way of saying that he was spiritual and *not* made of matter.

All the things that God created are mental, and never are, nor become, material. God's ideas are spiritual thoughts in contradistinction to a mortal's perishable thoughts, which are without substance and fleeting.

All God's thoughts are eternal, real, the substance of man's true individuality, and the essence of all created things. The entire panorama of *existence* from its first concept throughout its eternal unfoldment is, and ever will be, wholly mental—or, if you wish, spiritual.

It is only when man wrongly interprets the truths of being that he finds his lot, as Job had said,

"of few days, and full of trouble."

But when the first faint rays of enlightenment begin to dawn upon the horizon of his darkened consciousness, he will then learn what Plutarch had discovered nearly two thousand years ago:

"A man's felicity consists not in the outward and visible blessings of fortune, but in the inward and unseen perfections and riches of the mind."

CHAPTER XI

THE MOST disconcerting of all mysteries to man is death.

He cannot understand, if God is truly merciful, tender and loving, why he and his loved ones should become diseased, suffer and die, and frequently under the most painful circumstances. Nor can he equally understand what profit there can be in living a true Christian life if one must quite often succumb in the flower of youth, and in the greatest distress, while an impious and worthless fellow may live on in sound health to a ripe old age and expire in the peacefulness of slumber.

And, more, his perplexity eludes all sense of reason whenever he is reminded of these terse but oft-repeated statements from the Master:

> "This is life eternal! . . . If a man keep my saying, he shall never see death! . . . Whosoever . . . believeth in me shall never die!"

What then is it, he asks himself, that dies?

Merely your belief. A physical *sense* of death. Nothing else.

Death is an illusion. It is not true, because God never made it. It is simply a termination of the error that life is mortal. Death is as illusory as any disease and discord that thought can transform into health and harmony. God's man *never* dies.

So long as you believe that you are constituted of matter, you are compelled by the laws of matter to carry out this misapprehension of reality all the way to its terminus, a material sense of death. This is the nature of physical sense. And that is all that is physical, a *conscious* sense of yourself and your surroundings. Everything that is not real, or God-created, inevitably destroys itself. The only thing that can die is a mistaken apprehension of anything, the body included.

To keep Jesus' *saying,* or to *believe* in him, as he exhorted us to do, is to understand and demonstrate his teachings. Nothing more. Substituting worship of him for understanding the truth which he taught is to display spiritual ignorance. God alone should be the object of our worship, as He was the Master's. There is but *one* Deity.

This, Jesus himself confirms:

> **"The Lord our God is *one* Lord."**

If the kingdom of God is within man, as Jesus declared it was, and flesh and blood cannot inherit it, according to Paul, then it should be obvious that a physical form is not man, God's image and likeness, in which His kingdom abides. The physical form, erroneously called man, is an illusion, and exists in the mind of the one conceiving it; and this is what dies, a belief only.

Your real self, or individuality, is eternal. It can never be injured, nor can it die, since it exists in the mind of God. It is in His mind that you eternally dwell, notwithstanding the fallacious physical evidence that tells you otherwise.

Believing that you are a material entity, and self-contained, is the error which Jesus declared,

"is a lie, and the father of it."

Let us endeavor to consider this picture of God's kingdom with greater clarity. The fact that only an erroneous belief in man's mind is all that dies, particularly when a loved one or a best friend is laid away, can become downright bewildering to anyone not thoroughly instructed in the truth of being. A brief recapitulation, therefore, should conduce to bringing forward the desired light to this picture.

Everything that God had made, including its substance and structure, exists mentally—or, if you like, spiritually—in His mind. That is all there is, God's mind, in which are all the ideas which He has conceived, including man, you. There is *nothing* else. These ideas are His thoughts, and they are substantial and eternal. The whole is His creation. Man, being one of these ideas, can exist nowhere but in the Mind that conceived him. Space and time, hardness and softness, color and density, the moon and a Kansas wheat-field, are but a few more of His ideas. A bow and arrow, sight and sound, and the flight of a bumblebee, likewise are His ideas.

So are the flowing of a river in Brazil and the circulation of blood in your veins. None of it, the water, blood, nor activity of either, is material. All of it is simply a manifestation of God's mentality. His ideas remain ever the same, perfect, good and eternal, and never alter into any other form or substance from their original concept and pattern.

There is not so much as a split atom of matter anywhere in God's whole creation—or, if you wish, outside of it. Incidentally, there can be *nothing* outside of His kingdom. All that which appears to you as being outside of yourself actually is *within* you.

Where then, the question poses itself, is this apparent matter that we see all around us, including that which we have been led to believe constitutes our bodies?

The answer is, unequivocally, in our minds.

The materiality that we see everywhere is a mistaken sense of substance. Instead of seeing God's ideas as they have been created and forever exist, mentally, in His mind, we see a misconception of them, clothed in matter, and projected in *thought* outside of ourselves. This physical externalization is merely a deceptive belief in our consciousness.

Both pictures, God's true creation and man's misconception of it, are mental images throughout.

From time immemorial we have come to believe that we, and everything else that God has created, are material. And it is of this specific error, which has enslaved humanity with discord, want, disease and death, that the Master had declared:

"Ye shall know the truth, and the truth shall make you free."

The greatest of all sins is to believe that man is constructed out of material components, notwithstanding that you are unaware that there is no such thing as matter. All the faculties of spiritual cognizance which God has given him, mortal man expresses physically.

Paul's affirmation, that

"Ye are *not* in the flesh, but in the Spirit,"

cannot be repeated too often. And, by the same token, *nothing* else is, or can be, constructed of a physical nature.

Man is solely a mental idea living and having his being in God's mind, and constituted with every characteristic of his Creator. This is the image and likeness of God. *Everything* has its abode in His mind.

God's consciousness is His means of communication with all that which He has created, as it is the means of communication between the infinitude of ideas themselves. The whole creation, including all activity, growth, color, symmetry, unfoldment and purpose, is the kingdom which He perpetually reflects through consciousness to His offspring as their ideas of thought.

Man has no other means of communication with either God or His ideas, and this interchange of mutual interest can only be appreciated by mentality in furthering the ends of a purposeful existence.

When man multiplies, for multiplication is part of God's design, the kingdom is indivisibly correlated to *all* His offspring through this same conscious reflection. And notwithstanding the multiplicity of His image, each is an innate beneficiary, in consciousness alone, of the *one* complete and perfect kingdom. All this involved activity is everlastingly being manifested within the mind of God.

To illustrate: let us say that you are one of the images embraced in this multiplication. You cannot be a separate entity from God any more than a single ray of sunlight can go off by itself and remain separate from the sun. Actually you have no mind of your own, but rather are you the image or reflection, in consciousness, of God's mind. You merely coexist with your Creator as the sunlight coexists with the sun. You are amenable to God at all times. If this were not so, you would be nonexistent.

In other words, if God were to withdraw from existence this instant, you and everything else—from a cast-off stick to the planet Jupiter—would simultaneously disappear into nothingness.

You inherently are the reflection of *all* that is in God's mind, and in turn express that part of which you are aware. Acquiring and expressing more understanding is becoming increasingly aware of more of God's ideas. In this reflection, which is *you,* are all the other images of man, such as your wife, brothers, sisters and friends, and all those with whom you will come in contact in the future, inasmuch as they exist in God's mind too.

This is confirmed by the Master, thus:

> **"Before Abraham was, I am."**

This passage applies to you, too, no less than to Jesus. And it will dawn more clearly on your thought when you begin to realize that *all* of us, including the Master, are *one* with God, and have been so since the stars sang together at the cradle of creation.

The gaining of true knowledge, or understanding, is continually becoming aware of, and discovering, more and more of God's ideas and their peculiar functions. All that is, or ever can be, already is crystallized in the Creator's mind.

Solomon substantiates this fact:

> **"I know that, whatsoever God doeth, it shall be for ever: nothing can be put to it, nor any thing taken from it. . . . That which hath been is now; and that which is to be hath already been."**

You, conversely, are *in* the respective reflections that are the identities of all the other images, your wife, brothers, sisters, friends, and those with whom you have yet to make contact, for they similarly share *all* that is in God's mind, which inevitably must include *you*.

This should not seem incredible to you, that your wife, brothers, sisters and friends—yes, everyone and everything —are *within* you. Jesus made this quite clear, when he said:

"I am *in* my Father, and ye *in* me, and I *in* you. . . . That they all may be one; as Thou, Father, art *in* me, and I *in* Thee, that they also may be one *in* us . . . even as we are one."

All this activity, it is well to again remind you, is the unerring mentation ceaselessly going on in the mind of the Creator. God's offspring are but reflections—in consciousness—of Himself and His intelligence, as a mirror reflects your physical likeness and actions before it.

To turn back momentarily a thousand or perhaps a million generations ago, when our forebears became enmeshed in error, symbolic of the tree of material knowledge from which they were forbidden to eat, everything that basically was spiritual began to take on in consciousness a physical appearance. Of course it was only an illusion, to be sure, still these distant ancestors, such as they were, became gradually disposed to accept, and believe in, the reality of this deceptive phenomena.

It may have been a gradual metamorphosis, or a sudden one; its degree of mutation is of little consequence. But that which is of profound importance is the fact that it eventually became solid conviction, until today we have a crass materialism that seems virtually inextricable.

In the days of a greatly forgotten past, such oracles as Moses, Solomon, Isaiah and Jesus, among others whose influence still is with us, endeavored to enlighten the benighted mind. The Master, for one, said of those listening to him at the seaside:

"Hearing ye shall hear, and shall not understand; and seeing ye shall see, and shall not perceive; for this people's heart is waxed gross, and their ears are dull of hearing, and their eyes they have closed; lest at any time they should see with their eyes, and hear with their ears, and should understand with their heart, and should be converted (to the truth), and I should heal them."

It will of course be asked: from where did this first error, matter, come, if God's creation is a perfect one?

It came from nowhere.

Inasmuch as God's kingdom is a perfect one, and there can be none else, it should be self-evident that there is *no* place from which error could come. Consequently, it is an illusion, a misapprehension.

This seems perhaps an illogical, if not an absurd, answer at first thought; but by putting yourself in a corresponding position to a question approximating the one at issue, the picture clarifies itself at once, as for example:

"From where does the error come that says the sun moves around the earth once in every twenty-four hours?"

When you become aware of the truth that the sun is stationary, and that it is the earth turning on its axis every twenty-four hours that gives the deceptive *appear-*

ance of the sun in motion, you do not squander time probing for the error. Your acquired understanding of astronomy, limited as it may be, attests the fact that the sun moving around the earth is an illusion, a misapprehension of the truth. God's perfect idea, the science of astronomy, has no place for illusion.

So it is with *any* error, whether it be a misapprehension of the truth of being, a mistaken identity, or a false assumption or belief.

Bearing its own kind, after its own seed, your progenitors bequeathed you a pseudo-mind schooled in the materialism of the forbidden tree of knowledge.

And so it is that, while your heart wrings with grief as a loved one or best friend is being laid away, you see a mental picture of matter that appears external not only to your mind, but to all his other loved ones and friends in whose minds he similarly appears. What they buried in the ground was not the true individuality of this loved one or friend, for he always will dwell intact—as before—in the mind of God, but a physical misapprehension of this true individuality. In other words, they buried the misapprehension, the illusion, an erroneous belief.

What they buried was as devoid of actual matter as is the temple of their own minds in which he moved. The ground they laid him in, together with the rites performed at the grave, were in their minds. And when the assembled group of mourners returned to their respective homes, heavy of heart and slow of step, this, too, was part of the ever-changing panorama unfolding within the sanctuary of their minds.

The incredibility of the assumption that a material germ is capable of harming and killing the image and likeness of God, and mortal man to bury him, should of itself be enough to dispel the belief that man and the universe are material. One might as well attempt separating his reflection in the mirror from himself as to isolate God's image and likeness from His presence.

Dr. Alexis Carrel uttered a far more significant truth than he may have first suspected, when he said:

> **"Man is a stranger in the world that he himself has (materially) created."**

He can hardly be otherwise, living as he does in an illusory world of material phenomena. So long as he believes matter to be the substance of things, so long will he continue to stumble in darkness until swallowed up in the end by the grave.

That the belief of matter is the greatest of sins, and the strength of this sin is the intensity of your belief, Paul confirms:

> **"O death, where is thy sting? O grave, where is thy victory? The sting of death is sin; and the strength of sin is the law."**

Your belief that matter is real gives it the power of law which, in turn, chains you to the pillories of your own thought. You can free yourself of the terrors of this law, among them death, only in the degree that this destructive sin—your erroneous belief—is shorn of its strength by the light of truth.

Speaking of death and the invisible world, his eminence, John Henry Cardinal Newman, said:

> **"Our souls, when they depart hence, do not cease to exist, but they retire from this visible (material) scene of**

> things; or, in other words, they cease to act towards us, and before us, through our (material) senses. They live as they lived before; but that outward (material) frame, through which they were able to hold communion with other men, is in some way, we know not how, separated from us, and dries away and shrivels up as leaves may drop off a tree. They remain, but without the usual (material) means of approach towards us, and correspondence with us. . . . There are two worlds, the visible and the invisible."

God had created but *one* world, *one* kingdom, and the visible world which Cardinal Newman observed is but an illusion of it. The invisible, or real, world is invisible only to the material senses. The invisible world *always* is visible to your consciousness, else you could not so much as misapprehend it, see its illusion, the physical counterpart. It would be like looking into a mirror and seeing no reflection. Indeed, the invisible world is *not* made evident through an illusion of it. Such a belief is absurd.

God's man *never* held communion with other men through physical means. This is the misapprehension of spiritual man, this outward frame that appears to dry away and shrivel up as leaves may drop off a tree. And as for the soul, it does not retire from anything; but rather is it the belief of a material body, an illusion, that retires. There is but one possible explanation for matter: it absolutely does *not* exist.

Paul was unusually explicit on this point:

> "Look not at the things which are seen, but at the things which are not seen: for the things which are seen are temporal; but the things which are not seen are eternal."

There you have the clean-cut answer to the whole question pertaining to matter.

Let it not be inferred by this passage, however, that you do not see the things that are invisible. Nothing could be farther from the truth. Paul merely implied that the invisible, or real, is not apprehended by the material senses. Spiritual sense alone can cognize it.

If matter were real, why would you be told not to look at it?

What God made is spiritual; and if it were not actually seen by His offspring, or witnesses, what purpose or logic would there be to His creation in the first place?

Spiritual things *are* seen, emphatically so, and Paul sweeps aside all uncertainty on this point, thus:

"The invisible things of Him from the creation of the world are *clearly* **seen."**

It is only that your material sense of things, which is an erroneous sense, cannot perceive the actual substance of spiritual or invisible things. These are cognizant solely by spiritual sense, the only real sense that you have. If material sense could cognize spiritual sense, it would no longer be material sense. Our true sense is mental, *never* material.

So it was that Paul said:

"We walk by faith, not by (material) sight."

The life which you believe has departed from the body of a loved one or best friend was his consciousness, his only real entity. But this consciousness, or life, *never* in fact resided in his so-called material body, even when that body supposedly was alive and active. Rather did this material body in life, like the reflection in the mirror, symbolize this consciousness as an externalized thought.

What died was not the individuality of a loved one or best friend, for his consciousness alone was that individuality, or the real man, and this is deathless. Nor could a material body die, seeing that there is no such thing as matter.

It was merely his erroneous thought of himself that died. A belief in death.

That is all that ever dies, the externalized thought which we believe to be a verity, and to exist outside of ourselves. Nothing *real* can die, whether it be man, beast, tree, or one of God's eternal laws.

You are in reality a spiritual being carrying about an illusory material carcass.

Everything—man, animal, vegetable, mineral—appears as material substance because you observe it through the lens of physical sense, in your own mind. You do not see through the lens of a material eyeball for the reason that there is no material eyeball actually. This physical phenomenon is simply the belief that the real or spiritual eyeball, which is a component of the spiritual image, is matter.

To be more explicit, what you really see appearing physically are your own thoughts. Nothing else. And your *conviction* that these thoughts are material objects, external to yourself, is the substance of their solidity.

Anything that cannot entertain thought, cannot appreciate sight, hearing, feeling, taste and smell.

Inasmuch as the assumed *material* body of a loved one or best friend is but an externalized thought, nothing else, this explains why disease and all discord must similarly be the result of the same objective thinking.

Whether you realize it or not, you exist solely as consciousness. Your belief that you live in a material body is merely a projection of thought on the screen of your mind. Moreover, the present state of your body's well-being is the present state of consciousness which you are entertaining about it *in* this selfsame mind.

Your spiritual body, the image and likeness of God, which has form, density, color, symmetry, beauty and activity, is wholly a mental body, and this is your real individuality, your *only* individuality. Everything of necessity and interest is expressed within it. It lives on through all eternity, and you cannot possibly reverse or stay its purpose.

This is God's law, and

"It shall be for ever: nothing can be put to it, nor any thing taken from it."

Were this not so, you might perhaps desecrate, pervert or even destroy it, as the belief in matter inevitably desecrates, perverts and destroys most everything it assumes to be physical.

Fortunately this power is not put in the hands of a mortal, or illusory, entity.

Jesus was aware of God's law, when he said:

"The Son can do nothing of himself, but what he seeth the Father do: for what things soever He doeth, these also doeth the Son likewise."

You can see what the Father does only in your *consciousness,* and it is here that you repeat the action likewise. You merely reflect the power and identity of the kingdom *through,* and *in,* the medium of consciousness. The only thing you actually can destroy is your own errors, or externalized thoughts of matter.

Isaiah clearly states:

"For my thoughts are not your thoughts, neither are your ways my ways, saith the Lord. For as the heavens are higher than the earth, so are my ways higher than your ways, and my thoughts than your thoughts."

Man cannot desecrate, pervert and destroy God's thoughts and ways with his own, for mortal man's thoughts and ways are illusory.

Let us not delude ourselves that this thing we call consciousness is of our own making, that mortal man has the power of perpetuating it through his belief of a physical body. We simply are the reflection of God's consciousness is all. This reflection is His image and likeness. God is the matrix of everything that expresses Him.

If you are disposed to believe that real life is dependent upon physical phenomena, you cannot possibly escape its involvement in discord, disease and death.

Paul makes this clear:

"For I know that in me—that is, in my flesh—dwelleth no good thing. . . . So then with the mind I myself serve the law of God; but with the flesh the law of sin."

Nothing convulses man more than the apparent inevitability of death, notwithstanding that Paul and the Master, among others, have emphasized the fact that life is eternal, and there is *no* death. However, by believing in death none the less, man has given seeming reality to an incubus that is purely nonexistent.

Life for him can be little more than a relentless mockery, particularly when he still clings by instinct to the sustaining Infinite.

It is only by understanding the truth of being that disease is transformed into health, and the sting of death becomes powerless. This inspiring truth reveals the fact that your body is not constituted of matter, but solely of consciousness. It reveals also that it is your mind that sees, hears, feels, tastes and smells. And, too, it brings forth the conviction that everything you do, and the things with which you avail yourself to do it, is mental; and, moreover, that every deed and act is one of God's ideas being objectified, not as matter, but as thought.

Such understanding is precisely what Paul inferred, when he said:

"Death is swallowed up in victory."

It is well to keep this *ever* in mind: where your physical body seems to be is your spiritual body, visible only to consciousness. This body is the image of God, having outline, depth, form and color, and is eternal.

This is the body that you believe is material, but your belief is an *illusion*. Consequently, this illusory body that you have misconceived to be matter is, in turn, contaminated by this selfsame material thought with disease, and ultimately with death; and there you have the picture of what had died. A belief without existence.

In short, if your body was not spiritual, there would be nothing existent to be aware of a physical one, any more than your image could be reflected in a mirror without you standing before it. The reason for this is simple: there would be nothing to misapprehend, to misconceive, to be in error about. It is this misapprehension, this misconception, this being in error about, that is the *illusion* of a body that does not, and cannot, truly exist.

On her seventy-sixth birthday, Helen Keller said:

"I do not feel any age yet. There really is no age to the spirit."

The famed Miss Keller might well have appended to this truism:

"Nor is there death."

CHAPTER XII

MAN'S GREATEST concern in life is his body. His belief that it is matter precludes him from ever understanding it. And the further belief that his mind dwells *in* this body, rather than the body resides as a mental image in his mind, has enmeshed him in an entanglement of error from which he can never hope to extricate himself, except it be through a realization of the truth.

God's ideas are visible to your consciousness, and this is the only vision you have. They are your ideas by reflection, as you are His child by image and likeness. Ideas, whatever their identity, are no less image than is your individuality. They are images of awareness, in your mind, and nothing else. Were these ideas invisible to you, you would have absolutely no means of identifying *anything*, and creation therefore would be a vacuum to you.

To believe your body is matter is to admit that God is matter, if you are His image and likeness. But such a premise obviously is an error of illusion, for it is self-evident that God is Spirit and man His derivative, thereby making His offspring spiritual in substance. And what is spiritual fundamentally must be mental throughout God's entire design of existence.

That this is so, together with the fact that the material

body—like the spiritual—is equally a state of mind, Paul
corroborates:

**"For the mind of the flesh is death; but the mind of the
Spirit is life and peace, because the mind of the flesh is
enmity against God."**

There should be no question, according to the apostle,
that *all* is in mind, and therefore mental. There is no matter, and it is solely the belief of it in a carnal state of mind
that is enmity against the Creator, who knows nothing
of it.

The fact that your body is God's mental image assures
it of being a perfect body, assuming God is perfect, which
He admittedly is. Nothing can be added to this body, nor
can anything be taken from it. It is a complete body, and
does not lack any quality. It is ever the expression of perfect life, happiness, health, abundance, purity, satisfaction. This body can *never* vary a jot from its perfect state,
inasmuch as it exists in God's mind, and not as a substance called matter.

Consequently, it is an immortal body, because it exists
as a state of divine consciousness.

Your realization of this mental body is its spontaneous
activity. God always is manifesting it for you, feeding and
clothing it with His ideas. Your belief tells you that your
strength is in your physical muscles, that the senses of
sight, hearing, feeling, taste and smell are similarly in,
and of, this selfsame physical body. But this is a misapprehension of their true source. Your strength, sight, hearing,
feeling, taste and smell are rather manifestations of God's
image in your consciousness. They are not physical, but
mental.

Concerning your physical body, Paul said:

> "Whilst we are at home in the body, we are absent from the Lord. . . . We are confident and willing rather to be absent from the body, and to be present with the Lord."

To be present with the Lord is to see yourself, and everything else that He had made, in its true light, the substance of His mentality.

Your body is a state of consciousness. Its present state of health and well-being is your present state of consciousness. It is made up of God's ideas and more or less of your erroneous beliefs, such as being constituted of matter, and subject to disease and death among other things. Hence, in the ratio that God's ideas supplant these erroneous beliefs will your body become more perfect; while, conversely, the opposite is true when you misinterpret His ideas as being constituted of matter.

The Master exhorted:

> "Be ye therefore perfect, even as your Father which is in heaven is perfect."

There is no possible way for this state of perfection to be attained except it be through a transformation in your thoughts.

Everything you do is mental. Every act is an idea being objectified. It can never be objectified in matter, since there is nothing existent that is material. It is merely your thought that is objectified. Your God-given body has outline, solidity, form and color, but it is visible only to your consciousness. There is nothing else that can perceive. Your misapprehension of this God-given body is an objectification of it in matter in this selfsame consciousness, which erroneously believes *all* spiritual things to be material.

Your purpose in life is to be God's witness, His representative. It is your sole business to give evidence of the Creator, to express Him, for your individuality *is* this evidence and expression of Him. Your real self, God's image, is your identity *with* Him. You *are* His presence.

God's unfolding idea of man is the beating of his heart, the functions of his stomach, the kidneys, lungs, liver, and the perfect coordination of the whole. Constant realization of this divine law, without any material interference, will conduce to the continued harmony of these activities. The belief that you can improve God's idea, man, with matter, interrupts this harmonious continuity and provokes the seeds of doubt and fear, which eventually externalize themselves in disease and discord.

The desirability for perfection in man has been emphasized from Moses on down through antiquity to Jesus, and the latter's exhortations on this attainable goal have rung with the same assurance given us by the great Hebrew lawgiver, who declared:

"Thou shalt be perfect with the Lord thy God."

Your body is a perfect body, and this perfection is revealed only in expression. It is God's design to be expressed, consequently no part of your body should be suppressed. It is solely by entertaining a false belief about your body, or part of it, that suppresses it. To know that you *always* are capable of perfectly expressing God's idea, your body, will destroy the belief of suppression.

The vitalizing quality of your body is to become more and more aware of God's unfolding ideas. This unfoldment is the stimulus of life. Its discernment gives substance and vigor to your body. It is the essence and inspiration of your oneness with God, the animating power of your body.

The real body is without material parts. All of it is one part. It is perfect because it is God's image of Himself. It is His knowledge of Himself. It is *all* spiritual, hence mental.

Sickness is a material belief about this body, and actually it has nothing whatever to do with God's image and likeness. Pain is another phenomenon of this material belief. They can only evolve themselves in the *illusion* of God's image, the *belief* of a material body.

There is no more life within your material body than in the ten, twenty or fifty pounds of excess flesh which you chose to take off through diet. Were you to take off *any* additional amount, you still would be what you are. Any fatal effects occurring as a consequence of this performance would infallibly be the result of your own antecedent thoughts. Nothing deleterious can touch the real, or spiritual, body, and there is none other.

Healthy thoughts beget a healthy constitution as surely as diseased thoughts beget a diseased one, and this the immortal Shakespeare etched into the pages of true knowledge:

> **"For 'tis the mind that makes the body rich."**

Your body manifests inspiration because God's idea inspires. So does it manifest perfect assimilation, circulation, generation and elimination, all for the same reason. Too, it multiplies itself, in image, through procreation, because it is the law of God's idea to procreate. But only in Spirit,

Mind, does it do this, never in matter. Every function of the divine idea is your own function unfolding itself for your appreciation, satisfaction and delight.

Your stomach digests because God's idea unfolds digestion. To experience indigestion is to believe that the stomach digests of its own will. Indigestion is simply the phenomenon of the belief that the stomach is material and reduces matter to chyme. God's idea of digestion *must* digest, unless you have interfered through ignorance with His divine enactment by thrusting in the laws of material belief.

Paul makes this clear:

"With the mind I myself serve the law of God; but with the flesh the law of sin."

The law of sin is the belief that a material stomach has intelligence to digest matter and chemically prepare it for assimilation. And, by the same token, it implies also that the imperfect activity of your body, or part of it, is the result of the same belief that the flesh animates it. This explains the source of a stomach upset called indigestion.

By reflection your mind thinks, your kidneys eliminate, your heart beats with unlabored motion, all because God is doing this. He is reflecting to human consciousness His infinite love, wisdom and harmony. As matter, material phenomena knows *nothing* of what is going on. It can know nothing because it *is* nothing.

There is no pain in the body that is God's image. Pain is a belief *in* a body that does not really exist. Both the pain and the assumed physical body reside solely in the *mind* of the person experiencing the pain.

Should anything about your body appear to be out of

order, seek the perfect image of God in your mind, and *know* there is nothing in this spiritual body that can be disordered. You have no other body; and, as a result, the disorder will disappear from your experience proportionally to your conviction and steadfastness in this truth. The fact that your thinking can transform you in this manner is a divine law, and operates as such to both the belief and its phenomenon.

By clearly seeing this truth and convincing yourself that there is nothing really to get rid of, the belief loses its potency and disappears in the ratio to its dissolution in thought.

God perpetually reflects His love to you. But your belief that this love has ceased being reflected makes the belief of its suppression begin to manifest itself. And though this belief of suppression claims to exercise a nullifying power, it cannot actually nullify or give phenomena to anything, seeing it is without reality.

Paul substantiates this fact:

"There is no power but of God."

God does not nullify a single law in His unfolding creation; mortal man alone does this through his illusory belief of a material kingdom.

Only by understanding your body as a conscious idea, in God's mind, can you begin to understand God. Every fibre of your being expresses the sovereignty of the Creator. Thinking, knowing, evidencing, understanding, are His faculties, and these, among others, He reflects to His image and likeness. These infinite faculties are *constant*, because they are His eternal vision, or knowledge, of Himself.

The fact that God sees is the reason why your sight is eternal and beyond any possibility of accident. What God sees is what you see, and that is everything that He has created. These are His ideas, visible as images, or real objects, in your mind. Everything God had made is visible, but only in consciousness.

Seeing such things as He had *not* made is to see merely your own erring beliefs. These beliefs are illusory, materially-clad misconceptions of their spiritual counterparts. They are without substance or breath of true existence. They are lies, every one, the antipodes of God-created ideas.

The belief that the faculty of sight is material is to believe there can be imperfection in this faculty, which in itself is self-destroying. Its concomitant error, blindness, is believing that God's perfect idea of sight is not apparent in consciousness.

Had Jesus believed the erroneous evidence of matter when accosted by the two blind men imploring to be healed, surely he could never have said:

"According to your faith be it unto you."

But the Master knew, infallibly, that faith, sight and consciousness are spiritual substance, the substance of thought alone, and that there is positively no matter anywhere despite the deceptive appearance of it. Hence, the two blind men had but to attune their thought to faith, and thus were they healed.

Had Jesus believed otherwise, he would have stood on the same plane of conscious helplessness as the two distressed creatures whom he had succored. But he *knew* unquestionably that they were merely lacking in spiritual understanding, and it was in this understanding that he raised them accordingly.

Eyes as matter do not see. Eyes exist solely as idea, and are one with God's image. As matter they see nothing, know nothing, *are* nothing.

To illustrate: what becomes of the sight that once was assumed to be in the eyeballs of a corpse?

Obviously, nothing. It remains exactly where it always had resided, in God. It *never* was in the body that is this corpse, even when it was up and around. Material sight is as much an illusion as is the corpse in which it supposedly existed. God is your sight, your intelligence, your life, your body.

Sight requires no material channels. The belief of matter merely uses your consciousness to produce phenomena *within* the belief. It is all part of the grand illusion of a material existence.

Your nerves, as matter, do not feel. They similarly exist as idea. Paralysis is the phenomenon of the belief that nerves are lengthy material filaments, and have sensation within, and of, their physical structure.

God creates and gives existence only to His ideas, and needs no material channels to impart them for the purpose of His design. He is constantly reflecting Himself through consciousness, and this reflection is the whole pattern of His kingdom which is *within* you.

Your faith in God, that you *are* this reflection, is your protection from all evil. It is your assurance of perfect health, of contentment, of *everything* which you may possibly desire to this end.

Jesus confirms this:

> "Seek ye first the kingdom of God, and His righteousness, and all these things shall be added unto you."

Do not be afraid of your body, nor try too hard to understand the why and wherefore of it. The understanding will come with God's continual unfoldment of it, provided of course that you sincerely seek and strive for such understanding.

Come gently into this truth of the Spirit by waiting patiently for His *still small voice* to enter into your consciousness. For it is in your consciousness that your body resides, indestructibly, contentedly, eternally.

Paul exhorted:

> "Know ye not that ye are the temple of God, and that the Spirit of God dwelleth in you? . . . Let no man deceive himself. If any man among you seemeth to be wise in this (material) world, let him become a fool, that he may be wise. For the wisdom of this (material) world is foolishness with God."

The spiritual man's substantiality transcends physical comprehension, and therefore must be understood through a higher discernment than a material belief. And in the degree that God's universal idea replaces the false belief that you and the cosmos are constituted of matter, in that ratio will you react with a better and more perfect body. Such is the regeneration that takes place in your consciousness when truth begins to efface the deceptive appearance of a material creation.

Your individuality is realizing what God knows of Himself, and this realization is the reflection which you are.

Indeed, God will supply you the light to discern His kingdom if you but inquire after Him. Without realization, even in its most superficial application, all would be vacuity. The clearer that you see this reflection, or His image and likeness, the more distinct will become the outline and substance of your own individuality in your consciousness.

Any aspect of being clearly perceived tends to bring more vividly into focus the reflection of God which you are. You can know the *truth* only by identifying yourself with it.

By identifying yourself with matter, you take on the opposite characteristics of truth, or error. And from this misapprehension of true being arises the various discords of disease, pain, discontent, privation, and the like, which you experience. You are, in short, what you think.

Abandon your material *sense* of things; that is to say, abandon the belief that anything is made of matter. By doing this you do not abandon the thing itself, but rather the material *sense* of it.

The deceptive material thing, whatever it may be, has a counterpart in spiritual reality, in your consciousness, and surely you would not abandon that. Nor could you. This is God's idea, and it is indestructible. This idea, or image, *is* the reality of the thing in question, and it has its existence only in your mind.

Any appearance of this real image that invests it with matter is merely an illusion. And this illusion is the material *sense* that you would abandon. All of it is the process of mentation, or the conceptual activity of your mind.

Your whole purpose in life should be a constant seeking for, and the assimilating of, the divine character. This

alone will mold and fashion you anew, and bring you into
the glory and power of His likeness.

Paul expressed it this way:

**"Put off the old (material) man with his deeds; and put on
the new man, which is renewed in knowledge after the
image of Him that created him."**

You are the reflection, or image, of God's consciousness,
nothing more nor less. This reflection is His kingdom, and
it is your function to express it. It is *all* done mentally.

If you would revitalize and make perfect your body, you
must constantly be discovering that it is quite different
from the one which you had heretofore supposed it to be.
You must continually look *for,* and *at,* your body in God.
It is in no other place. It is simply a mental reflection in
your consciousness. Your sight, smell, taste, hearing and
feeling, similarly are in God, and are solely mental, or
spiritual, as is your body.

By looking to God for health and strength, you will
surely find it. By looking for it in the illusion of a material body, you will find only the kindred errors of this
illusion, which are disease, pain and death.

Ralph Waldo Emerson well said:

**"We must get rid of all thought of self before we can gain
peace or happiness."**

This *thought of self* is to believe that your individuality
is *in,* and constituted *of,* matter; and its conviction is im-
prisoning yourself within the outline of this very belief.
Indeed, this thought of self is the most pernicious of *all*
erring beliefs in human experience to get rid of.

Yet such riddance is the momentous step one must take

in the spiritual transformation that will make you anew.
Summing up the matter, Paul declared:

"**They that are after the flesh do mind the things of the
flesh; but they that are after the Spirit the things of the
Spirit. . . . The mind of the flesh is enmity against God:
for it is not subject to the law of God, neither indeed can
be. So then they that are in the flesh cannot please God.
But ye are *not* in the flesh, but in the Spirit.**"

CHAPTER XIII

WHAT IS faith?

Many notable figures from time immemorial have attempted to answer this modest question, but none perhaps has interpreted it more clearly and simply than the Hindu ascetic, Mohandas Gandhi, who said:

"Faith is nothing but a living, wide-awake consciousness of God within."

Ponder well these words of wisdom by this mighty religious leader, and nurture them daily with your thought so that such a faith may establish itself firmly in your consciousness. No one can truly know what faith is until it is experienced in some degree by the recapturing of health, contentment, peace of mind, or through discovery of divine law.

The rewards from a great faith can be almost unbelievable to our intellectual grasp. The ends of true achievement come only through faith. It is the motive power of existence.

Jesus said to the diseased woman:

"Thy faith hath made thee whole."

And she was made so from that hour. The Master made it plain that it was her *own* faith that healed her.

This should not be difficult of belief, that one's own faith can overcome any diseased condition or disorder, for Jesus emphatically declared:

> "What things soever ye desire, when ye pray, believe that ye receive them, and ye shall have them."

To live graciously, contentedly, healthfully, agelessly, is to live by faith. A living, wide-awake consciousness of God within is our soul going out to Him for all that we desire. This is the light that illumines our way in the dark. It is patience and self-reliance.

Daniel sharing the lion's den without fear of harm was a demonstration of this living, wide-awake consciousness of God within. So was the faith evidenced by Shadrach, Meshach and Abednego who were cast into the fiery furnace without so much as their hair being singed. Similarly was the Master's performance of walking on the water without sinking such a faith. While a mother's simple prayers to God in the small hours of the night that healed her sick child also testified to this living, wide-awake consciousness of God within.

The Apostle James said:

> "Every good gift and every perfect gift is from above, and cometh down from the Father."

This fact, that every good gift cometh down from the Father, is the inspiration for the faith that discovered, developed and perfected such ideas as the electric dynamo, phonograph, sewing machine, automobile, radio and television, among a host of other inventions. Faith is the impulse that incited the thought which brought forth their realization.

Were the kingdom of God *not* within you, there would be neither purpose nor reason for evidencing faith. The affinity which the kingdom of God has for faith is beyond human comprehension. It is this correlation one for the other in spiritual consciousness that expresses man's unity with his Maker most profitably. Without faith there would be no incentive to gain the divine ear.

St. Augustine said:

"Faith is to believe what we do not see; and the reward of this faith is to see what we believe."

Faith is power. It is tremendous power. Notwithstanding that it is an invisible power to the material senses, it is clearly visible to your spiritual sense. Faith is demonstrable in any situation, and an abiding trust in God will surely bring this power into your daily experience.

Entertaining the faintest fear or doubt diminishes both the quality and strength of your faith. Conversely, to confidently *know*, with resolute conviction, that you are *one* with God and constantly coexist with Him, is to be in perfect rapport with its design and unfoldment.

Faith evolves the things in life which we desire for fulfilling the ends of our purpose. Were these things not already established within us, faith would be powerless in bringing them into realization. But the fact is incontrovertible that everything *is* in us, in our consciousness, if the kingdom of God is within you and me, and the desert nomad wandering across the desolate Sahara.

Paul said it this way:

"Faith is the substance of things hoped for, the evidence of things not seen. . . . Through faith we understand that the

worlds were framed by the word of God, so that things which are seen were not made of things which do appear."

So simply stated is this passage that it utterly dethrones matter once and for all as being real substance.

The two blind men that followed Jesus, crying after him that he have mercy on them that they might see, were moved by the conviction that the Master could heal them; and Jesus, having compassion on them, gently touched their eyes, and said:

"According to your faith be it unto you."

And their eyes that moment were opened.

It is well, at this point, to ponder over the brief statement that the Master had made. Observe that he said to the two blind men, "according to *your* faith," for herein lies the great secret of spiritual potency.

Unless your *own* faith is great enough to equal the problem to be overcome, neither Jesus nor anyone else could be of avail to heal you. The chemistry of all healing is faith in your *coexistence* with God, and therefore in the perfection of *all* that He had made, including yourself. This is the measure of your sincerity and devotion to Him.

Jesus knew that the kingdom of God was within these two blind men, if in a dormant state. Consequently, it was plain to him that he had but to lift their faith *accordingly;* and, lifting it thus, this loftier realization of Truth's power healed them.

Neither medicine was dispensed nor was there need of a scalpel to perform a delicate operation on matter. It was simply faith alone that healed them. And it was all done in a moment.

Indeed, it was not Jesus' faith, which admittedly was great enough, but their own that restored their sight.

The contrary is likewise true when there is *no* faith, as when Jesus returned to his home town, and was there looked upon with disdain, being as he was the son of a carpenter. According to Matthew:

"He did *not* many mighty works there because of their unbelief."

Jesus himself substantiates this Biblical record. In answer to these townfolk who were offended in him, he said:

"A prophet is not without honor, save in his own country, and in his own house."

Nevertheless, Jesus well *knew* the power that comes to one who leans on God alone. He said:

"If ye have faith . . . ye might say unto this sycamine tree, be thou plucked up by the root, and be thou planted in the sea; and it should obey you."

The power of faith evidencing itself in your experience, whether it be put to the capacity to heal, or simply to achieve complete peace unto the soul, will be in the ratio of your conviction that man and the universe are not material, but spiritual. If the sycamine tree can be plucked up by the root and planted in the sea by a mere command, as Jesus had pointed out, then everything in the creation is undeniably mental in substance, construction and activity, and therefore the entire unfoldment of existence must be solely a manifestation of Mind.

By the widest stretch of the imagination the sycamine tree could never be material, actually.

And why should this be incredible?

Did not the Master say:

"Whosoever . . . shall not doubt in his heart, but shall believe that those things which he saith shall come to pass; he shall have whatsoever he saith."?

If the kingdom of God is within you, and you have dominion over it, it becomes rather obvious why the things you ask of yourself should come to pass. Your thought, your consciousness, *is* the kingdom.

However, it would be impossible to have absolute faith either in yourself, or in God, so long as you harbor the faintest semblance of doubt or fear in your heart.

Materiality can never benefit from the fruits of faith, because there is *nothing* material in existence. Faith has affinity only for the spiritual, seeing that spiritual consciousness is all that is real. Spiritual consciousness is the substance and intelligence of yourself, the image which you are of God. It is the substance and power of your faith.

The Master said, on another occasion:

"Ask, and it shall be given you; seek, and ye shall find; knock, and it shall be opened unto you: for every one that asketh receiveth; and he that seeketh findeth; and to him that knocketh it shall be opened . . . and all things, whatsoever ye shall ask in prayer, believing, ye shall receive."

When your faith rises to meet the demands of your desire, God's gifts come to you without fail, in spiritual consciousness. There is no other existence nor receptivity that can possibly be aware of His infinite blessings.

Therein lies the beauty, grandeur, stability, perfection and holiness, of creation, this amazing fact that it is a manifestation in the mind of God. Man's erroneous sense of it can harm or destroy nothing but his own mistaken concept of it. This creation which God had made becomes the more marvelous and inspiring when we but realize that *all* of it actually is *within* us, to be utilized for our eternal joy.

O, what ignorance and darkness governs the minds of men that war and hate, and pursue after iniquity and avarice, and who have not love and charity and humility in their hearts!

Spoke the prophet, Malachi:

"Prove me now, saith the Lord of hosts, if I will not open you the windows of heaven, and pour you out a blessing that there shall not be room enough to receive it."

Think of it! The potential joys that are within your very possession, if only you will recognize their source, and the humble conditions by which they may be realized.

These blessings are all spiritual; they only *appear* material to our erring sense of the real.

CHAPTER XIV

PRAYER IS the solvent that clears away the mists of illusion from man's coexistence with his Maker.

Prayer is humility, an inward search of the soul, a sincere seeking of self-purification. It is to *know* with conviction that God is your identity, as your image in the mirror identifies your *own* personality. It is equally to know that He has provided for every perfect function of your body, from digestion to circulation. And, too, it is recognition of the fact that to believe yourself a separate entity from Him, and to fancy an affinity of your spiritual ego with matter, invites disease, pain and death.

Prayer is the realization that you are God's perfect child. It is the magnetic attraction drawing you ever closer to Him. Constant and grateful acknowledgment of this glorious truth, as well as for the fruits which come from its understanding, enriches your prayer. And if you sincerely feel the yearning, the humility, the gratitude and love, which your words to Him express, He will ever answer:

"Son, lift up your face to Me! *Look!* All that I have is thine."

Eloquence, despite all its loftiness and euphony, is not prayer. It has no power to heal. The power is in the humble baring of the heart, together with the conviction that God will answer your petition. Prayer is a living, pulsating faith that your desires will be evolved for you notwithstanding your lack of rhetoric.

The qualifications necessary to demonstrate God's unerring healing power are sincerity of purpose, an intense desire to know Him, and the earnest aspiration to express His love. That you shall strive to be morally upright is imperative if you would manifest this healing truth.

To adapt yourself to these demands of divine law is prayer.

It is well to be reminded of Jesus' admonition, following his healing of the man that had been impotent with a burdensome infirmity for thirty and eight years:

> **"Behold, thou art made whole: sin no more, lest a worse thing come unto thee."**

It is obvious that good morals, honesty, and the unceasing expression of God's love, are as requisite to healing as they are prophylactic in their nature toward the inception of disease.

Woe unto him that would lessen these demands to conform to his own pattern of righteousness rather than to the divine standard!

To turn your thoughts away from the belief of a material body, and to see yourself as a spiritual idea in God's mind, is efficacious prayer. With this picture fixed distinctly in mind, talk to Him, informally, as you would talk to a friend, or your mother and father, for indeed God *is* your Friend, and your Mother and Father too. There is none other.

God will not only understand you, but His omnipresence will so inspire you with divine exaltation that a new world—the real one—will begin to unfold in your consciousness. All things will appear divested of their material composition, and their *real* nature and substance will be revealed, exactly as God had made them, and intended them to be appreciated.

It is said in Psalms:

"He that dwelleth in the secret place of the most High shall abide under the shadow of the Almighty."

This dwelling in God, perceiving everything forged in the substance of consciousness, while oblivious of it being molded out of matter, is a foretaste of the eternal life promised by the Master. Indeed, it is a far clearer perspective of the kingdom than that which is seen in the illusion of matter. All of it is the manifestation of the Creator's mind.

Your prayers should be for an increasing understanding of this divine unfoldment, rather than for material desire, which has no reality in fact. There is absolutely *no* material thing nor substance either inside or outside of God's kingdom. God knows of nothing cast in matter. He reflects His ideas to you spiritually, without need of a material intermediary, through consciousness alone, and the abundance of these ideas are far more than you can begin to comprehend, much less utilize.

Instead of praying for health, be grateful that you always have been the reflection of God's *perfect* idea, and the mere realization of this truth in your consciousness will transform any disorder into the picture of health which you hold steadfastly in thought. Such gratitude is the essence of effectual prayer.

Dr. William S. Sadler reveals this interesting bit of information brought to light by medical research:

> **"Recently, in the clinic, we have most thoroughly tested the therapeutic value of prayer. We have been astonished to discover the wide range of functional disorders, physical disturbances and psychic difficulties, which have been wholly cured or greatly helped by this simple procedure; and, to our utter amazement, some of the most remarkable cures were effected in the case of patients who frankly told us, at the time we prescribed prayer, that they did not believe in praying, that they did not have faith in God."**

Prayer is dynamic power when sustained by faith. Without faith it is impotent. This is God's law. His idea. Long-winded declamations in the praise of His grandeur, wisdom and mercy are ineffectual in so far as bringing about an improved state of health, or conducing to harmony where discord prevails. Such verbiage may serve the ends of pompous solemnity, but it will not heal the slightest disorder. Prayer, combined with a deep but sincere faith, needs no verbiage, and will fulfill *any* desire.

Prayer, amply blended with the potency of faith, is the alchemy which prompted Jesus to say:

> **"With God all things are possible."**

God's proximity to you is in precise relation to the distance in which your thoughts place Him. The closer you bring your coexistence with God in thought, the more faithful will your experience in life pattern His perfection. Harboring positive thoughts will draw Him ever nearer to you as surely as negative ones will obscure His presence. Inasmuch as God's kingdom is exclusively a mental domain, within your consciousness, all power obviously is vested in your thinking.

Make it a habit to affirm at frequent intervals the fact that God's presence always is within you. Remind yourself, too, that His presence is the substance of your individuality. Begin to lean more on Him, so that He might guide your footsteps. Put your problems before Him, as you would put them before a counselor or confidant. Ask for His advice, then trust Him with all your heart, with all your soul, and with all your mind.

This is true prayer. This is having atonement with Him. At-*one*-ment. And if your sincerity of heart is half equal to the determination with which you seek Him, He assuredly will answer you.

Said Lord Tennyson:

"More things are wrought by prayer than this world dreams of."

When you pray to God, do so calmly. To believe that you can reach Him through emotional or desperate frenzy is to instantly make inoperative the unfoldment of prayer. Nor is it efficacious to beg Him, as one might beg of a human being. God is not moved by beggary.

Prayer is simply giving voice to your faith, and faith is the antithesis of emotion, desperation and beggary. Faith, as Jesus has set forth, is to believe with all your heart and soul that that for which you ask will be forthcoming. The whole process of prayer from beginning to end, from desire to fulfillment, is in your consciousness. It is part and parcel of the kingdom of God that is within you. Your faith is the balance that tips the scales in prayer.

Professor William James said:

> "As regards prayer for the sick, if any medical fact can be considered to stand firm, it is that in certain environments, prayer may contribute to recovery, and should be encouraged as a therapeutic measure."

You yourself must make this *certain* environment. Environment, like everything else that God has created, is mental. It exists wholly within your own consciousness.

If prayer excites the power to heal in some instances, surely it must be the divine remedy in *all* instances. Jesus proved this incontrovertibly.

To prepare yourself for the power that heals, you first must make a spiritual atmosphere in which only you and God are present. This state of propinquity is not difficult to establish; it already *is*. You need but to sweep away the cobwebs of matter from your consciousness to perceive it. Indeed, there can be nothing else present in the entire universe but you and God.

You and God include the *all* of omnipresence, seeing that you are *one* with God. By the same token, if His kingdom is within you, it is obvious that *nothing* else can possibly be present.

Therefore, you create this desired atmosphere with the only medium available, your spiritualized thought. Spiritualized thought is simply appreciating everything in your mind as God had actually made it, and intended it to be perceived. All of it is devoid of matter, devoid of material structure. This is the way the true picture must be discerned. It is *all* mental, from concept to unfoldment to fulfillment.

It is well to set aside brief intervals daily when you can be alone with God, even though these intervals last but a minute or two, or five, or longer. Relax yourself completely. Close your eyes to all material surroundings, to all phenomena of matter, and rather dwell upon their true counterpart in the sanctum of your consciousness. This is the only place they can, or ever did, exist.

Jesus specifically alluded to this effacing of all phenomena of matter, when he said:

"When thou prayest, enter into thy closet, and when thou hast shut thy door, pray to thy Father which is in secret; and thy Father which seeth in secret shall reward thee openly."

This passage implies coexistence of Father and son, that *all* is Mind, that matter is illusion, and that the Father hears and answers prayer in and through consciousness only, the sole agency by which His image can gain His attention.

Being constantly aware of these truths is the quality of prayer to which the Father is responsive. It is losing yourself in His presence, moving about mentally in the infinite breadth of His mind.

Incidentally, it is your *real* individuality moving hither and yon, for it is self-evident that no physical personality could thus be at large in Spirit.

Paul clearly confirms this:

"In Him we live, and move, and have our being."

Increase your mental visits with God. Drink deeply of
His wisdom and power. Imbue yourself with His inspiration. Feel your *oneness* with Him permeate every fibre of
your being. And, in good time, you will begin to experience a transformation gradually come over you that will
be little short of astounding.

This is making for yourself a spiritual atmosphere. It
is the certain environment indicated by Professor William
James. It is the environment that unerringly *heals.*

Richard Chenevix Trench, Archbishop of Dublin,
clearly interprets the ineffable exaltation of such an environment:

"Lord, what a change within us one short hour spent in
Thy presence will avail to make! What heavy burdens
from our bosom take!"

If you would enter into the quintessence of pure prayer,
live among your fellow men as if God were one of them,
and observing your every action. And, too, converse with
Him at all times as if these same fellow men were present
and giving heed to your every word. Then you will be
living your prayer rather than making use of it occasionally
as a means for living.

To live such prayer one must conscientiously strive to
observe the injunction set forth by the Master:

"Love thy neighbor as thyself."

Man will have come a long way in his search for truth
who practices this simple admonition.

Perhaps the greatest use made of prayer is in behalf of the sick and dying, and this is easily understood. It was through this ailing condition in mankind that Jesus undertook to prove the works of God. Prayer heals *all* disorder.

Robert Burns, the Scotch poet, had well said:

"They never sought in vain that sought the Lord aright."

Man generally turns to God when all material means of assistance have been expended. Indeed, God should have been his *first* recourse. This extremity in which he finds himself, however, offers God the only bona-fide opportunity to manifest His omnipotence. Deep down in his heart, man is not unaware that there exists some inscrutable tie that correlates him to his Maker.

Nothing proves so clearly the futility of matter, when likened to this bond with God, than human suffering and the imminence of death. Too frequently is prayer, considered in the light of physical belief, like the proverbial straw to which a drowning man clings.

There is this remarkable difference, however: prayer, when accompanied by the smallest measure of faith that you are *one* with your Creator, will do what the straw can never hope to accomplish.

That this is so, Dr. Alexis Carrel verifies:

"As a physician, I have seen men, after all other therapy had failed, lifted out of disease and melancholy by the serene effort of prayer."

And then, amplifying this disclosure, this famed medical practitioner and Nobel prize winner adds:

"Our present conception of the influence of prayer upon pathological lesions is based upon the observation of patients who have been cured almost instantaneously of various affections, such as peritoneal tuberculosis, cold abscesses, osteitis, suppurating wounds, lupus, cancer, etc. . . . This proves the objective importance of the spiritual activities, which hygienists, physicians, educators and sociologists have almost always neglected to study. They open to man a new world."

This illuminating declaration by the distinguished surgeon and member of the Rockefeller Institute for Medical Research is but one more of the countless testimonies of prominent medical scholars disproving the curative powers of medicine. And, too, it also refutes the false statements circulated by many of his colleagues in the practice of medicine that the alleged healings resulting from prayer, or other forms of divine faith, have restored merely psychical or emotional disturbances rather than functional and organic diseases.

Obviously, these misleading utterances, voiced for the sole purpose of combating the rapidly-growing trend toward spiritual, or metaphysical, healing, have been the precursors to the introduction of psychosomatic medicine.

These material errors have been pointed out, every one of them, by the foreknowledge of the Master:

"By their fruits ye shall know them."

Every honest physician knows that prayer and faith in God to heal, brief though his service in the profession might be, have restored to health the diseased and disabled, who only grew worse under medical treatment. Few turn to God unreservedly before first depleting the nostrums of at least a half-dozen specialists.

Dr. William S. Sadler, recognizing the mighty influence of prayer and the forces of Spirit to heal, declared:

> **"More than half of the present afflictions of mankind could be prevented by the tremendous prophylactic power of the Christian religion. . . . Some day the world may awake to the point where it will recognize that the teachings of Christ are potent and powerful in the work of preventing and curing disease."**

Who then is so presumptuous to say, in light of such authoritative testimony, that man's faith in God, rather than in medicine, cannot heal him of disease?

St. James said, succinctly:

> **"The effectual fervent prayer of a righteous man availeth much."**

St. James was simply stating that the deep and heartfelt prayer of anyone resolved to live according to the highest precepts of good, or God's law, surely will be answered.

Jesus put it even more to the point:

> **"What things soever ye desire, when ye pray, believe that ye receive them, and ye shall have them."**

To look deeper into the gist of the matter, prayer is merely an avowal to your conscious self that you are *one* with your Maker, and that you dwell eternally and in perfect health and harmony in His mind, as His mental image. *Everything* exists as mental image in His mind. Actually you are as close to God in this *oneness* as an image of your own thought is *one* with you. Image always is *one* with whoever conceives it, whether it be God or you. It is this affinity that engenders divine healing.

The purpose of scientific prayer is not merely to acknowledge this perfection and harmony which you are, and let it go at that, for this would avail you nothing. It is rather to vividly *see* and *feel* yourself perfect and harmonious. Such sight is not physical; it is purely mental. And in the ratio that this perfection crystallizes in your consciousness, and the imperfection about yourself disappears therefrom, will your prayer be answered.

Paul brings this out clearly:

"Are ye so foolish? having begun in the Spirit, are ye now made perfect by the flesh?"

God already had made you perfect when He created His kingdom. You cannot be otherwise, although you may appear so to yourself in belief. It is this illusory appearing, which you yourself have outlined in your thought, that you must transform into perfection and health—in your consciousness—through the medium of *truth*.

It is God's law that gives you the power to bring into focus your perfect state of being through this transformation in your thinking. Your part is solely to administer this law and set it into action through realization, for realization is divine activity. The innumerable ideas that are yours to be conceived and profitably employed only *seem* encumbered with matter.

Charles Proteus Steinmetz, a giant himself in the conception of these ideas in electrophysics, said:

"I think the greatest discoveries will be made along spiritual lines. Some day people will learn that material things do not bring happiness and are of little use in making men and women creative and powerful. Then the scientists of the world will turn their laboratories over to the study of God and prayer and the spiritual forces which, as yet, have hardly been scratched. When that day comes, the world will see more advancement in one generation than it has seen in the last four."

To trust God with our problems, even the intimate secrets that lie hidden within the darkest recesses of our hearts, is the most wholesome tonic that can be prescribed for the anxiety in men's souls. Its salutary influence allays the torment of both an abased conscience and the plight of mental imprisonment; while, at the same time, it cleanses the mind of all undesirable beliefs and replaces them with the stimulus of God's ideas.

Take God into the fulness of your confidence. Dwell constantly on Him. Know that everything good and profitable is His idea, and that it is solely these ideas which you utilize in consciousness that bring about the ends of your individual purpose.

Know, too, as the Psalmist had declared:

"It is God that hath made us, and not we ourselves."

Always keep in mind the fact that there is *no* place you can be that God is not there. You can never be alone, for His presence ever envelops you. And, more, be assured that you need never fear anything, knowing as you should that He is steadfastly protecting you from all harm.

Such thoughts are efficacious prayer.

Trust God with all your heart. Lean heavily upon Him. Let His wisdom guide you. And, above all, hold steadfastly to Him notwithstanding the seeming odds against you. For in the degree of your cohesion to Him will that tranquillity of mind come to you which is beyond all understanding.

This, too, is prayer, and the most availing kind.

If you truly desire to seek God, with all your heart and with all your strength of mind, and with an abiding faith that you coexist with Him—not materially but spiritually— then will Isaiah's prophecy surely unfold,

"And thine ears shall hear a word behind thee, saying, this is the way, walk ye in it."

William Ewart Gladstone, distinguished British statesman and Liberal leader, asked what kept him so serene and composed in the midst of his busy life, gave this reply:

"At the foot of my bed, where I can see it on retiring and on arising in the morning, are the words, 'Thou wilt keep him in perfect peace whose mind is stayed on Thee, because he trusteth in Thee.' "

These words of Isaiah confirm the fact that *mind* alone is the actual substance of your being. Your faith that God's evidence of Himself is unfolded within this selfsame mind brings out more clearly His kingdom that is within you.

Your prayers are never presented in vain, except they be clouded with doubt, fear or insincerity. Somewhere, sometime, if only you will listen patiently for that *still small voice* of Omnipotence, your humble petitions shall be answered.

It is as the poet, John Masefield, had said:

"God warms His hands at man's heart when he prays."

Whenever the sick, the lame, the blind, the deaf and the impotent, pray to Him with all their heart, and with all their soul, and with all their strength of mind, unwaveringly and with patience, God will unfold to them *the miracle that heals*.